STETHOSCOPE
on REALITY

How My Journey as a Working-Class Jew from
Brooklyn Informed My 50 Years of Medical
Practice, Opening My Heart and Mind

ERIC LESSINGER, MD

Fulton Books
Meadville, PA

Published by Fulton Books 2022

ISBN 979-8-88505-374-7 (paperback)
ISBN 979-8-88505-375-4 (digital)

Printed in the United States of America

In memory of my many mentors, especially
Jacob Lessinger, my father, 1911-1987
and Harvey Jackins, the founder of
Re-evaluation Counseling 1916-1999.

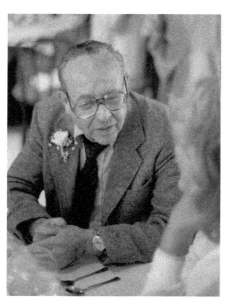
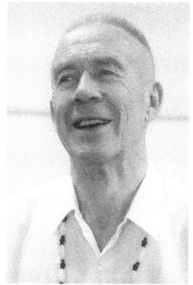

CONTENTS

INTRODUCTION

I graduated from the New York University School of Medicine in 1972. This book is a memoir of my life specifically in medicine, which of necessity includes the experiences which made me who I am. What I was taught, what I believe, and where I place my faith, as a working-class Jew and a human being.

My view of the world, from very early on, was strongly influenced by two related traditions in my family:

First were long-standing Jewish values:

Welcome the stranger. Strive for excellence.

Heal and repair the world.

Second were the ideological underpinnings of the political left, as I understood them:

Strive for a better economic and social system, so that people could be kind and fair to one another, and so that there would no longer be such a very large gap between rich and poor.

I am a second-generation American. My mother's parents were poor. They were born in Eastern Europe, and each of them came separately to America during their late teens, to escape the pogroms. Arriving at Ellis Island by boat, they initially settled on the Lower East Side of Manhattan, where immigrant Jews and Chinese were concentrated at that time.

My parents were working class. My father went to City College in New York at night, to earn a Bachelor of Business Administration degree. My mother went to college for one year. I became the first and only medical doctor in the family, although my brother and most of my cousins also went on to get higher degrees.

In those days, many Jewish families were eager to move out of the traditional working-class jobs, and to be "upwardly mobile," at least in the sense of social class. They became professionals, such as teachers, social workers, and doctors. And although there was still rampant anti-Semitism, there was also an opportunity to pursue the path of "upward mobility." My brother and I did just that, and very successfully so. From New York City public schools, both my brother and I went to Harvard College on full scholarship. At Harvard I met owning class people for the first time, but I didn't really get to know many of them. The Students for a Democratic Society (SDS) became my social and political home at Harvard. I was eager to live in a better world, and

I believed that it was possible. That belief is even stronger now, toward the end of my career. I believe that capitalism has outlived its usefulness, although I can't claim to foresee what system would replace it. From Harvard, I went on to NYU Medical School, which did not display the same snobbishness as Harvard but presented difficulties of its own.

My beliefs and activism broadened out in medical school. As SDS started to fray politically, I could not find a political home among any of the three factions (which were Revolutionary Youth Movement [RYM I], the Revolutionary Youth Movement II [RYM II], and the Weathermen). We formed a group locally in New York City calling itself the Movement for a Democratic Society, which had a committee focused on health, but it didn't last long. The NYU administration was none too happy with our small radical crowd in medical school either. Students from several medical schools formed the Student Health Organization (SHO), which was decidedly left-wing, despite its neutral-sounding name.

In my final year as a medical student, I was able to arrange a clinical rotation for two months on the Navajo reservation in Arizona. That was an eye-opening experience. It also touched my heart and kept me thinking about medicine, oppression, and the possibility of real social change. When I graduated from NYU in 1972, I got my MD degree.

I did my internship year at Lincoln Hospital, in the South Bronx. When that year was completed, I got my NY State license to practice medicine.

I was eager to start practicing medicine as soon as I got my license. I looked for a practice opportunity, and I found one in Rochester, New York. I was competent enough to practice, but I also knew that I would want further training as a resident.

Family practice, as distinct from general practice, had just become a specialty. I went on to get fully certified as a family physician and proceeded to certify in the subspecialties of geriatrics and hospice and palliative care. I spent the last twelve years of my practice working exclusively in hospice and palliative care. Those years provided me with many of the most memorable and rewarding moments of my medical career.

SECTION 1: FAMILY

My first few years at home

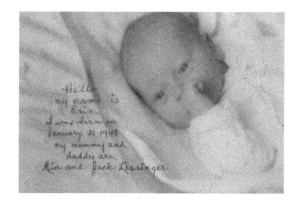

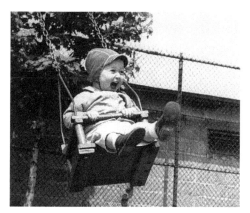
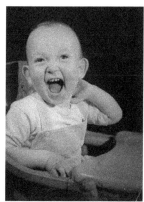

I was a happy kid.

I was born in a hospital in Brooklyn, New York, on January 31, 1948. When my mother was pregnant with me, she was healthy, and I suspect that life in the womb probably felt good to me. Obviously I couldn't have had any information which might have helped me understand what was going on in the world outside. As I reflect back on it now, I have reason to suspect that my mother was frightened. I believe that I may have picked up signals that she felt scared from stress hormones that transferred from her circulation to mine. That, in turn, might have scared me.

What was going on in the world at that time? My mother had given birth two years before to my sister Karen, who was severely disabled, and whom my parents placed in an institution, with great sadness. I was growing and developing just fine as a fetus inside my mother, but my mother couldn't know that for sure, not knowing whether I would turn out like Karen. I suspect that I picked up on that fear as well. Also, my parents were communists. The Soviet Union, which had been our ally against the Nazis, was now our arch enemy. And the true horror of the Holocaust was still coming out to the public. Israel was declared a state in 1948, the year I was born.

My birth went well; I was healthy, and I seemed to be happy from very early on.

My parents were loving and kind, and they tried to follow the child-rearing advice of the time, largely that of Dr. Benjamin Spock. I can remember only one time that I could hear fear in my father's voice. That was when I heard him arguing downstairs with an FBI agent who showed up at our front door. I was only about six years old at the time, but it has stayed with me as a vivid memory, at least emotionally.

Grandma and Grandpa Kalish

From the time that I was born until the time I was in third grade, my family lived with my mother's parents, Fannie (née Fega Horowitz) Kalish and David Kalish.

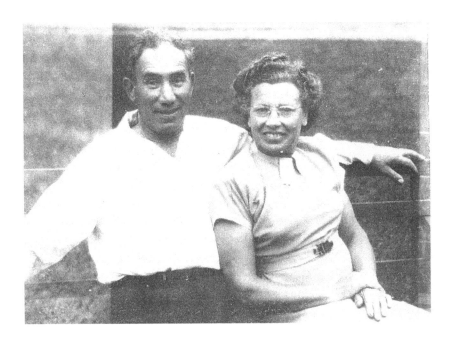

They were both born around 1889 in the Pale of Eastern Europe. David lived in a shtetl near Ostropol, in Ukraine. He worked as a carpenter or carpenter's apprentice there. (When my family lived with him until I was eleven years old, he would teach me carpentry skills, and his praise consisted of telling me, "Now you're a half a carpenter!") The

1880s were a decade of pogroms, when Cossacks would ride into town on horseback, to burn, loot, rape, and kill. To escape all this, in 1905, David walked nine hundred miles to Hamburg, Germany, where he would board a ship to America, at age 16.

Fannie also grew up somewhere near Ostropol. Her father worked for a wealthy farmer as a book-keeper, and she did chores even as a young child. Milking had its benefits, though, especially drinking off some cream. She developed a fine head for numbers, helping her father with the books. She did the same for the business which she and her husband David later owned in Brooklyn. She fled across Europe alone, also at age sixteen, traveling mostly by train until she reached Liverpool, whence she sailed alone across the Atlantic Ocean until she reached New York City and was welcomed by the sight of the relatively new Statue of Liberty, as well as the poem at its base. ("Give me your tired, your poor, your huddled masses yearning to breathe free, the wretched refuse of your teeming shore. Send these, the homeless, the tempest-tost to me. I lift my lamp beside the golden door!") That was a rela-tively accurate description of my grandparents' sit-uation when they arrived in America.

They arrived knowing no English. Yiddish was their first language. On the Lower East Side of

Manhattan at that time was a large community of impoverished Yiddish-speaking immigrants. Fannie and David were both put up by relatives who had preceded them to America. Their families introduced them to each other, and they married in 1907.

David heard that there were jobs in Detroit for workers with skills such as he had and that they paid relatively well. Having no children at that point, they left the poor community of the Lower East Side and relocated, where David worked at the Ford Motor Company. He got to be a skilled tool and die maker. During the First World War, he worked for the Cadillac factory inspecting tanks. The left-wing tradition in my family starts with my grandparents. Grandpa was a union organizer at a time when the bosses would bring in Pinkerton Agency guards to break up union meetings by breaking some heads. My mother was born in Detroit in 1913. Apparently, my grandparents were also ahead of their time in the area of family planning. They made babies in 1911, 1913, and 1915. Fannie went to a doctor for advice, and whatever they did, it worked.

Around 1930 they moved back to New York, where they became naturalized American citizens, and bought a home and store on Eighteenth Avenue in Brooklyn. It was a small row house, in a neighborhood called Borough Park. It was a working-class neighborhood evenly divided between Jews and Catholics. The neighborhood consisted of attached two-story buildings, and most of them had small shops on the first-floor storefronts; next door was a small dress factory with half a dozen seamstresses in back, and a dress sales shop in front. It was owned by an Italian Catholic woman. On our other side was a Jew, Mr. Adler. At Mr. Adler's candy store, he sold fancy and not-so-fancy candies, snack foods, and newspapers. (That's where I developed my taste for chocolate-covered Maraschino cherries). Grandpa would send me next door with nickel and two pennies. For him, he instructed me to buy a Yiddish newspaper thus: "If he's got the *Freiheit* (Freedom, the communist paper), buy that. If he's got the *Forverts* (Forward, the socialist newspaper), buy that. But if all he's got is that rag, *Der Tug* (The Day), don't bother!" For my two cents, I could get two pretzel sticks or one Maraschino cherry.

In Grandma and Grandpa's store, everything they sold was made to order—venetian blinds and window shades, glass for windows and mirrors, and wooden frames for the windows and mirrors. They would score and cut the glass themselves. Grandpa did most of this work; Grandma did some of this work; she also kept the books. She did all the housecleaning, food preparation, and cooking. Grandpa's contribution on that front was to ferment cucumbers in a yeasty barrel to make half-sour (*not* dill) pickles, and to steep dried sweet cherries in schnapps. Grandma Fannie's kitchen was where I developed my taste for chicken soup with kreplach, apple pies with lots of cinnamon, and matzoh brei (which she taught me to fry up for myself, eventually). Although Grandma undoubtedly did much of the intellectual heavy lifting in their household, I think Grandpa called the shots. I didn't think of this as male domination of my grandmother by my grandfather at the time. I certainly didn't understand it as such. Later, in my parent's relationship with each other, I became a little uneasy about the patronizing treatment of my mother by my father, but at the same time, my dad was my role model. And the rest of US society in the 1950s reinforced sexist attitudes fairly openly.

My grandparents' living space consisted of a living room, a kitchen, and a tiny bedroom off the kitchen. There was also a small backyard behind the house. The backyard was where Grandpa planted two fig trees, which he tended carefully, wrapping them in burlap to protect them from the winter climate in the Northeast US. Every summer, they bore fruit, and we had the pleasure of eating fresh figs off the tree, which are very different from the dried figs you can buy anywhere now, although they are equally delicious. As I recall there was also a little tool shed and a makeshift fort where my brother Les and I would play. This magical place also held a small depression under a lilac bush, which we filled with a mixture of water and urine and soil and whatever rotting scraps we could find. This concoction was dubbed *doody brown*, and Les, whose favorite pastimes seemed to be making jingles and torturing me, would threaten, in a sing-song manner "My doody brown, you'll drink it down!"

My family lived on the second floor. We had a living room, a bathroom, and two bedrooms. Les and I shared a bedroom there, until we moved to another neighborhood when he was twelve years old, and I was eight. (There we each had a bedroom of our own). From the stairs near the back of the building, we would go through my grandparent's place to play in the backyard.

My grandparents survived through two world wars, epidemics of polio, smallpox, typhoid, and influenza, and the Great Depression. They both lived into their upper nineties, and their marriage lasted sixty-seven years.

Grandma and Grandpa Lessinger

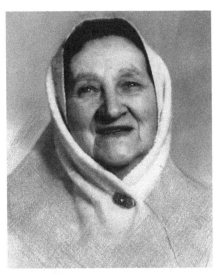

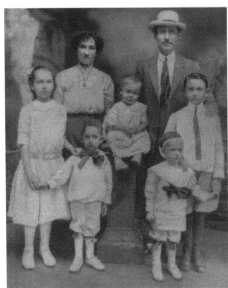 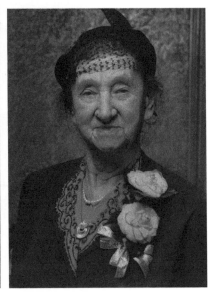

Nettie, Joseph, and their children. My father is
the youngest, shown between his parents.

I know less about my father's parents. They were already married when they came to America from Austria. Grandpa Joseph died when my father was young, so I never met him. I believe that he worked as a tailor, that he had a volatile temper, and that he was an observant Jew. When Grandma Nettie was widowed, my father had to go to work at an early age to help support the family. In the only formal portrait photograph of Grandpa Joseph that I saw, he cuts a dashing figure, wearing an elegant white hat and white suit.

I don't know where Grandma Nettie lived when my family lived in Brooklyn. I can't remember her visiting us, though she probably did, at least a few times. My strongest memory of her was when I, at age nine or so, went with my family to Penn Station in New York and watched her get on a huge silver train, moving to Aiken, South Carolina, to accompany her daughter Adele, who was going to marry a man named Sonny Wolff. I hadn't known that there were any Jews living in South Carolina. I don't remember seeing any of them again, but Sonny and Adele did have two children.

Grandma Nettie was devoutly religious. My father took a photograph of her draped in a white shawl lighting Shabbos candles. She also has a formal portrait photograph in which she looks very well-dressed, with a small black hat to which a lace veil was attached, covering her upper forehead.

My father was one of five children. They all turned out to be more conservative and religious than he. (The only supporter of Donald Trump in the family that I know of is one of my older first cousins. By way of contrast, one of my first cousins on my mother's side was named Eugene Victor, after Eugene Victor Debs).

Red-diaper baby

I always knew that I was a Jew. I am what is called a *non-observant*, secular Jew. Jewish culture was celebrated by my family; Judaism, or Jewish religion, was not. Belief in God was for the Catholic kids, who would say things like "Ooh, God is going to put a pimple on your tongue, because you told a lie!" No one in my family believed in God; no one talked about it. I later learned the term *atheist*. That is who I am, although *atheist* is yet one more identity which makes me *feel* less safe, on top of *Jew* and *Communist*.

I heard only English and Yiddish in my house growing up—no Hebrew. I did not go to Hebrew School. I went to a Yiddishe Shule (Yiddish School) briefly, taught by a man named Leib. My older brother actually *graduated* from Shule. Although I believed in the righteousness of our duty to heal and repair the world, I didn't know the Hebrew words for that concept (Tikkun Olam) until I embraced my Judaism more fully in my twenties.

I was thoroughly steeped in far left-wing politics, and I have remained so all my life. My parents were members of the communist party (CPUSA). Hence, I was a *red* while I was still in diapers. My brother and I, along with hundreds of other

Americans, were labeled *red-diaper babies*, and if we self-identified as such, we were proud of it.

My parents tried to protect me somewhat from the fears associated with being a Jew and a communist, but at the same time, they taught me a lot about communist tradition. Paul Robeson's rich bass voice was played on seventy-eight RPM records in our house; my father took many photographs of Robeson, including Robeson at the podium during the convention of the American Labor Party in 1948, held at a packed Carnegie Hall. I knew about Gus Hall, national chairman of the CPUSA, who ran for president of the United States four times, and Benjamin Davis, who actually served several terms on the NYC Council as a Communist, representing Harlem.

Then came the *red scare*. Very quickly the USSR went from being our wartime ally to being our enemy. Once the US unleashed the atomic bombs on Hiroshima and Nagasaki, Japan, a nuclear arms race began between the *superpowers*. It was not a shooting war, so it got dubbed the *Cold War*. Any American associated with communism was labeled a traitor. Numerous draconian laws were passed by Congress, often unanimously, such as the Smith Act, making membership in the party illegal. I believe that it is still technically illegal to be a communist in our country. But if the party still exists, it no longer poses any threat, and no one is prosecuted just for membership anymore. But in the 1950s, communist *sympathizers* such as the *Hollywood Ten* were fired from their jobs, and officers of labor unions were also stripped from leadership. Senator Joseph McCarthy even has an *ism* named after him.

And if being a communist wasn't enough, my dad was also part of a small group of socially concerned photographers called the New York Photo League, who I knew to be friendly people, and they occasionally met in our living room. They were labeled *communist sympathizers*, and they were also investigated. One couple from the league emigrated to England to avoid this madness in the US.

J. Edgar Hoover, head of the FBI, was in hot pursuit of *commies*. The House Un-American Activities Committee (HUAC) subpoenaed hundreds of witnesses. American communists were indicted and jailed for spying and perjury. Julius and Ethel Rosenberg were convicted of spying for our enemies, the USSR, and of selling them the *secret of the atomic bomb* (which turned out to have little real value, since the Soviets were close behind us in the development of the atom bomb technology anyway). They were sentenced to death, and they were executed on June 19, 1953, at Sing Sing

Prison in Ossining, New York, by electrocution. Smoke arose from their heads as the deadly current was applied to metal caps. My brother and I were only five and ten years old, but still, I was aware that something awful was happening. The Rosenbergs were Communist Jews, just like us, and they left behind two sons, Robert and Michael, ages six and ten. The orphans were adopted by a close family named Meeropol. There but for the grace of God go I.

My parents — Jacob and Minnie Lessinger

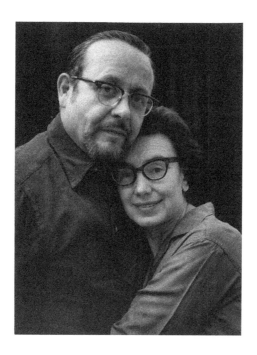

Growing up I lived with my maternal grandparents, my parents, and my brother. My sister had lived and died without us ever meeting each other. My grandparents influenced my sense of Jewishness, of class, and of politics, in a good way. My mother was their daughter, but given the sexism we all absorbed, I looked to my father for information about the world, and my mother deferred to him. Looking back, I now wonder also about how much the women in the family might have been leading, but not getting respect for it, nor acknowledgment of it. Grandma

Fannie kept the books for the business, and she did some of the same work as Grandpa David. She also did the shopping and the cooking. Maybe she was really the unacknowledged leader of the household.

My father, Jacob Charles Lessinger, was born on February 4, 1911, in New York. My parents met in New York, possibly when they were both at City College (CCNY), and they married young, on July 1, 1933. My father had some serious challenges as a young man. His own father, Joseph, died young, leaving my father to work in order to contribute to the family income. And my father developed a malignant tumor before he turned 30; a soft-tissue sarcoma on the top of his right foot.

The only available treatment at that time was amputation, and there were no internal prostheses at that time; only external. His surgeon removed his right foot, keeping a large flap of skin at the bottom of the foot to attach and fashion as a heel pad. He wore a specially made tubular cushion sock, into which he inserted a somewhat heavy external fiberglass leg with a regular shoe attached, which stayed permanently tied. With his pant cuffs pulled over it all, it appeared indistinguishable from a real leg and foot. He walked with a limp which came from a shortened but functional right leg. His leg was even shorter without the prosthesis.

My father didn't hide his amputated leg from me or Les—on the contrary, he would lie in bed on Sunday mornings and play with us by poking at us with his stump. However, his was a significant disability. He couldn't run or ride a bicycle, or play basketball, which he had done informally through high school and maybe even in college. He couldn't let the sock and prosthesis get wet, and it was too heavy for swimming anyway, so when he went down to the community dock in the summer, he would take off his prosthetic leg, and launch himself in a shallow dive off the end of the dock. As I recall, the young children stared at the sight, but after they got to a certain age, everybody looked away and pretended not to notice. I'm also remembering now, as I write this, that I was disappointed to have a dad who couldn't play catch or toss around a football with me. Some of my lack of serious interest in sports was related to this. Les, even though he grew to be well over six feet tall, showed essentially no interest in sports at all. He fit the description of *bookworm.*

My father's experience with surgery led to a life-long interest in all things medical. There was no social security or health insurance back then; he had no assets to speak of, nor did he have enough cash on hand to pay for such a large expense as an amputation. He and I never discussed it, but I suspect it was done at no cost to him, in part because an amputation in such a young patient was an unusual, if not unique, situation for the surgeon and the prosthetist. I do know that my father was pleased by the results of his surgery, and proud of his surgeon, Dr. Haagensen. He became famous as a breast surgeon, and wrote a book in 1956 which created a system for classifying breast cancer.

My father graduated from CCNY with a degree in business administration. This qualified him to become a certified public accountant (CPA). At some point, he went into business with a couple of his brothers, running a small store. He mostly did personal income tax returns at first, and then they added photocopying to the business at some point. It was a wet process (called photostats), copies took a couple of hours to develop.

Later still, my father took on a third identity, as a commercial and professional photographer. This really became his passion and his life's work. On the back of many of his prints is his rubber stamp: Jack Lessinger, professional photographer. He developed a vast collection of pictures over the years, mostly of people. Social justice was the main theme. Striking workers, Romani children on the street, workers in Portugal, informal portraits of dignified older black women, formal portraits of Dr. W. E. B. DuBois. I came into his entire photo collection and many of his papers when he died. He died on January 1, 1987, of his second heart attack, at age seventy-five.

My dad told me that he had written to some medical schools to ask whether he could enroll, but they advised him that he need not even apply, given his lack of the prerequisite course work, as well as being older than the typical medical student. Later, when he worked as a professional photographer, he came as close as he ever would to working in medicine, developing a professional relationship with an eye surgeon, going into the operating room with him and filming real surgical procedures through an operating microscope. He showed them to me before I went to medical school, and I'm glad that I was never squeamish, because some of those scenes of corneal transplants, and especially of buckle procedures to treat retinal detachments, were nasty! My dad didn't really have to push me into medicine—he modeled interest in it, and medicine surely fit the advice he gave me about what I should do with my life: do something that I was good at, and do something that was really needed in the world.

I don't know with any degree of certainty about the genesis of my father's commitment to communism. From what I know about my father's family, it didn't come from them. It seems that he would have to break away from their religiosity, their relative conservatism, and their middle-class pretensions to arrive at such a drastically different ideology. I think that his ideas must have changed when he lived with my mother's parents. Grandpa David brought his left-wing activism over from the Old Country. As a naturalized citizen, he had to declare on his papers that he was a *not an anarchist*. But he could read Yiddish, and the newspaper which he clearly preferred to read was the communist one. He went to Camp Kinderland in the thirties, which was a summer camp in upstate New York, founded in the 1920s by communists and union leaders from New York City, to allow their families to get out into the countryside, to promote left-wing politics, Yiddishkeit, and sports.

My mother, Minnie Kalish Lessinger, was born in Detroit, Michigan, on October 11, 1913. She went to City College in New York for one year. She worked as a secretary briefly. She married my father when she was twenty and he was twenty-two. Compared to her own mother, Grandma Fannie, my mother's role in the family appeared to be more circumscribed. She really deferred to my father. He even did a fair amount of the cooking. And even though she was clearly intelligent, I believe that she was never the same after my sister Karen was born.

My mother teared up when I first asked her about my sister. After Karen was born and made a ward of the State, my mom went to some other place in her own mind. I think that she couldn't bear to think about Karen. She had to keep telling herself that Karen never would have amounted to anything. Losing any child is hard. This might have been harder because Karen had been a girl, and my mother wound up living in an all-male household after that. My mother gradually became very hard of hearing, and also developed Alzheimer's disease. She needed assisted living and then skilled living in a nursing home. I brought her to Ithaca, and despite the injunction against treating oneself or one's family ("the doctor who treats himself has a fool for a patient!"), I acted as her attending physician at the nursing home until she died on December 2, 2010 at age ninety-seven.

My sister Karen

Sitting in my backyard in Brooklyn, the sky a perfectly cloudless blue, under the fig trees which my grandfather had planted, following the lines of the song, which promised that "every man 'neath his vine and fig tree shall live in peace and unafraid." I looked up at the branches, which bore the promise of sweet, soft, seedy fruit.

My cousin Gene and I were both young boys at that time. He was two years older. We were lazily passing the time, when he said, seemingly out of the blue, "Your sister died." What?

"I never had a sister."

"Oh, yes you did. My mommy told me. Her name was Karen."

I was totally shocked. I was not sure I should believe him, because he and my older brother Les used to play tricks on me sometimes.

I was the youngest of all the cousins on both sides of the family. I had never met, nor heard of, nor seen "Karen," even in photographs, and my dad was a professional photographer, who seemed to take pictures of everything and everyone, especially our family.

It didn't take very long to summon up the courage to ask my mom whether it was true. She got a dreamy, far-off look in her eye, and teared up at my innocent question. It was true. My brother was born when my mom was thirty. I was born when my mom was thirty-five. But in between, she had given birth to a girl, and they named her Karen.

Well, Karen was somewhat small at birth, and her face didn't look quite right. It soon became apparent that she was in fact not right. She didn't meet early developmental milestones, such as head control, and her cry didn't sound normal. She was *retarded*, but no one seemed to know why. She didn't have Down syndrome. Apparently taking care of Karen was challenging physically and emotionally, but mostly it was discouraging, even seeming hopeless. (At some point they did find out that she had congenital rubella syndrome, but that did not essentially change anything.)

As Jewish working-class parents in the 1940s, they had high expectations for their children. My older brother Les already seemed precocious in their eyes. He would likely become upwardly mobile in his social class position without much difficulty. But Karen, not so much. Caring for her seemed like it would be difficult, and she might soak up a lot of time and attention.

It seemed unlikely that anyone would want to adopt Karen. With some sadness, my parents decided to do something that was common at the time—they gave her over to the care of New York State. Willowbrook State School was a very large, overpopulated warehouse for badly damaged children. It later turned out that Willowbrook became the subject of a horrific scandal of criminal negligence and worse. I was told later that Grandma Fannie used to take the Staten Island Ferry out to the institution to visit Karen regularly.

Apparently, my parents, already taking care of one healthy baby, and feeling badly about the other, couldn't bring themselves to visit her. In fact, they literally cut her out of their lives. The only surviving picture which I have of her is a birth announcement, showing my parents and my brother, and apparently Karen as well, with accompanying text welcoming her: "There's a new arrival in the pee-pee and poo-poo department of the Lessinger household," but Karen's image had literally been cut out with scissors to show only my parents and Les as a two-year-old. Karen died at Willowbrook, of *natural causes*, at about age eight.

My mother's sadness was profound. I absorbed her sadness, and I felt confused. From her I heard a refrain which was to become burned into my memory, and which I heard many times thereafter whenever the subject of Karen was brought up: "She would never have amounted to anything anyway."

After the initial shock, my parents told me that since they had one healthy child, they felt ready to try to have another, and that child turned out to be me. My birth itself was a source of relief and a cause for celebration. I was more than eight pounds, I had a strong cry, and I seemed to develop into a happy child.

One other thing I have sometimes wondered about. What if things had been different? What if my parents had the support they needed, to raise Karen as one of the family, without sacrificing their ambitions for me and Les? Having one child who wasn't *going anywhere* socially or professionally, and who *never would have amounted to anything anyway*? It seems to me that Karen might just have provided our family with a calming tonic to our frenetic drive toward upward mobility.

My brother Les

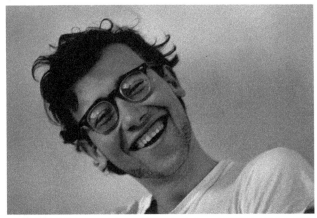

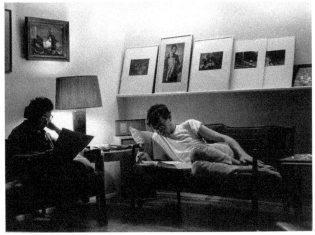

Leslie Lessinger was born on June 29, 1943 in Brooklyn. He was named after the famous British left-wing actor Leslie Howard, who was a bomber pilot in World War II, and who had been shot down and killed just before my brother was born.

Les was four and a half years older than I. We loved each other, and I looked up to him. Due to our age difference, we never actually went to the same school at the same time. But we did spend summers together. My family and my aunt Eve's family both bought small houses in a small community in Putnam County, one hour north of New York City. There were thirty families, and most had progressive political views.

My brother helped me out a lot. I have a photo of him on the community dock, helping me to bait a hook. The dock was used for swimming (and for fishing when there was no one swimming, in the early morning or the evening). When my family bought a small wooden row boat for fishing around the edges of the lake, we named it the "Leric."

He could also make life miserable for me at times. He teased me often; sometimes he would threaten me, although it was difficult to tell when he might be joking. Part of Les's experience growing up was stereotypically male—little boys were made of *snips and snails, and puppy dog tails*" I don't think that he tortured any animals, but he didn't like to take care of our pet dog Nippa any more than I did. (We gave her away after a little while). I previously mentioned his gleeful threat to make me drink *doody brown* in the backyard where we first lived (a foul-smelling liquid containing urine, rainwater, mud, and God knows what else). Some of the *jokes* I learned from Les were oppressive to various groups, and many had to do with bodily functions. Possibly the most benign which I can remember goes like this: "Ev'ry body's doin' it, doin' it; pickin' their nose and chewin' it, chewin' it; they think it's candy, but it's (s)not!"

I felt competitive with Les even though he was older. The selection of a valedictorian at Stuyvesant was determined solely on the basis of grade point average, calculated out to the tenths of points. I can well remember that Les's average was 98.4, while mine, four years later, was *only* 97.3.

I tried to do whatever my big brother did; I emulated Les in just about everything, even though I didn't always plan it that way. He married Hanna as soon as they graduated from Harvard/Radcliffe. I married Ellen as soon as I graduated from Harvard.

Les developed pancreatic cancer in his early sixties when he was living in Brooklyn. I was a hospice doctor living in Trumansburg, New York at that time. My experience with patients who had pancreatic cancer was not encouraging. The prognosis was grim. I had never known a patient to be cured. If that has changed, it may be that there are more effective chemotherapies now.

When Les was diagnosed, the only treatment was surgery, and I was leery of that, because I had never seen the surgery be curative, and also because the complicated Whipple procedure had major risks of its own, including a poorer quality of life. I didn't get to discuss it with Les and Hanna. His doctors did a Whipple on him, which removed the head of his pancreas and his bile duct and rearranged the way his intestines were hooked up. As I feared, although the CT scan showed no evidence of metastases at the time of surgery, micro-metastases must have been there in his liver, as well as in his pancreas, because he became jaundiced again in a few months. He had a feeding tube. He got sicker and sicker, and I don't know what his doctors were thinking at that point, but I do know that he was enrolled in a home hospice for just two days before he died.

I don't think that I could have changed the way his doctors treated him, nor that his death in 2010 at age sixty-seven could have been prevented. Once again, though, I am left wondering whether things might have been different. Treatment for many types of cancer is more effective now. But back then, the prognosis for long-term survival of pancreatic cancer was not good. Les was subjected to a serious surgical procedure, which seemed to me like a *Hail*

Mary attempt to beat the odds of his poor prognosis. This led to long-term use of a gastric feeding tube, which means, among other things, that you don't get to taste your food.

Perhaps less aggressive treatment of his cancer might have improved the quality of his life after the diagnosis of pancreatic cancer, and it might even have lengthened his survival. Even with such a rapidly moving disease, there should have been enough time for months of palliative care before enrolling in hospice. I'm not pleased with many aspects of medical care in this country, and I'm sad and angry about the care that Les was given.

Now, everyone from my family of origin is gone.

Section 2: SCHOOLING

Elementary school

I have vague memories of P.S. 48, in Bensonhurst, which I attended from kindergarten through second grade. When I was nine or ten years old, my family moved to Kingsview Cooperative apartments, at the corner of Myrtle Avenue and Ashland Place. The new neighborhood was Downtown Brooklyn. My local school was P.S. 20. I went there for grades three through six, and I remember it well. First off, I entered part way through the school year. I knew no one; most of the others had been there since kindergarten. Secondly, the neighborhood was very mixed; I would guess roughly one-third white, one-third black, and one-third Puerto Rican. Along Myrtle Avenue ran an elevated train, and on the other side of Myrtle Avenue from Kingsview was the Fort Greene Public Housing Project, which was huge, with forty-six thousand apartments, built after World War II.

It had all the ills of *the projects*—relative poverty, violence, and drugs (although there were few overdoses at that time). Kingsview, with fewer than six hundred apartments, was an early attempt at neighborhood "gentrification," which did not "succeed" until much later, long after I had moved out in 1964.

After my abbreviated third grade, I was put into a special *advanced* class, where all of the students stayed with the same teacher for the next three school years. My class picture from 1958 shows the teacher and only about twenty students (a smaller class than many at the time).

About half of the students were black, with a few Puerto Ricans. It was the first time I was aware of routinely seeing African Heritage people in person. There was only one boy in that class with whom I developed a friendship and he was a white Protestant. There were three people other than me in that class who also lived in Kingsview. I did visit those classmates outside of school, and I would sometimes meet with them in their apartments. There was no one else whom I saw regularly outside of school. In the class, there was one black girl who I could tell was obviously smart. My father told me that he knew her father, who was a leftist, and also an academic. But I had already absorbed the racist social conditioning which made me feel superior to all black people.

Our lives were quite segregated. The co-op where my family lived was overwhelmingly white. The Fort Greene Housing Projects across the street were crowded with poor black and Puerto Rican families, and I believed, true or not, that there was a lot of drug use and violence there. On the television was *The Amos 'n' Andy* show, who were two black buffoons who couldn't speak proper English, and their friend *Kingfish*, who was just as bad. Even the liberal Jewish writers of Broadway musicals, which I loved growing up, had unsubtle stereotypes in "Porgy and Bess," and "West Side Story." Back then, I knew very black people in positions of power, or who were treated with respect.

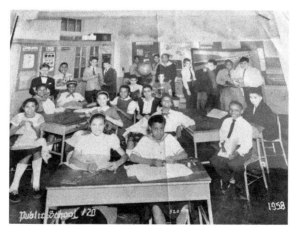

This photo of my sixth-grade class shows
Mrs. Farrar in the back, and me in a
jacket pointing to the blackboard.

I was also conditioned to feel superior to the girls in class, although I could tell that some of them were obviously smart. I never was encouraged by my parents to tease or abuse girls. I didn't see girls as if they were from another planet, or feel that they had *cooties*. We furtively passed notes back and forth, or *flirted*, although we were all pre-pubertal and innocent. All three of the girls who I thought were cute were white and dark-haired. There were four Jews in my class.

The teacher of this special class was Mrs. Evelyn Farrar. She was a black African Heritage woman herself, but I didn't recognize that about her at first. I think that there were several reasons why I didn't recognize it at first. She didn't fit the racist stereotypes which I had already absorbed. Mrs. Farrar didn't fit the images I had seen of black people on television in the 1950s, who were not teachers or anyone else in positions of power. In her speech, I heard no trace of the Southern US nor a Caribbean accent; her diction was clear and crisp—not the black English I heard on the street in the new neighborhood. Her appearance showed self-respect. She was probably in her forties, stood erect, and rarely smiled. Her hair was straightened, and it was pulled back into a bun. Her natural skin tone was brown, not black, and she wore a little bit of pink pancake make-up. When somebody told me she was black, I couldn't quite believe it. Here was a black woman teaching me! Once I accepted this as fact, it was just another lesson learned. I remember her as kind, somewhat distant, and a good teacher.

One very vivid memory I have of Mrs. Farrar is calling upon us in turns to come up to the front of the room, and to begin the day by reading a Psalm from the King James Bible. The first time I heard the 23rd Psalm, I was enthralled, and I have continued to draw strength and inspiration from it ever since. (You know, the one that starts with, "The Lord is my shepherd; I shall not want," and ends with, "Surely, goodness and mercy shall follow me all the days of my life, and I will dwell in the house of the Lord forever.")

Those Psalms are in my own Jewish tradition— Psalms of David. And even though such readings would no longer be allowed under separation of Church and State, I'm glad that I had the experience. Maybe all high school students should be required to study comparative religion.

On my last report card for sixth grade, Mrs. Farrar wrote to my parents, "Never have I seen such stick-to-it-ive-ness in one so young."

Early adolescence

Being twelve years old was not easy for me. I had been interested in girls for a couple of years already. I thought it gave me an advantage over the other boys in getting into relationships with girls—I had never gone through a period like other boys, when they thought that girls were somehow *yucky*. Some girls looked cute to me, and I was excited to realize that they were interested in me too. Outside of school, the neighborhood seemed too unsafe to visit my friends in their homes, whether male or female.

At some point, along with the other boys, my interest in girls became more intense. I was unaware even of knowing any young people who were attracted to people of their own gender (*gay or lesbian*), but I had absorbed the strong societal norms which disapproved of homosexuality at that time. And I really didn't like the way other boys talked about the girls. Lots of crude sexual innuendos.

I went through the usual physical and emotional changes of adolescence. I felt lucky that the pus pimples on my face were not any worse than they were. Some boys developed permanent acne scarring as they got older.

Living in my family, my brother and I were expected to be thoughtful and polite and in control. Like all Jews, we lived with some degree of fear, whether we were aware of it or not. We felt that we might be betrayed or even killed, as irrational as that was. My brother Les, being five years older, controlled himself, and he gave me the option of controlling myself, or being controlled by him.

I believe that every person can feel a full range of emotions, under appropriate circumstances. I certainly felt things, but for me it was easier to show the feelings of fear or sadness, not anger. (This is still true about me, even today.) One time in the late evening when I was twelve, I couldn't contain my anger. A few years later I couldn't even remember what set me off. Everyone else was home, so I closed the door to my room, turned off most of the lights, and started attacking my blanket. I used a large pair of scissors to slash it soundlessly again and again. I did feel a little better after the catharsis of the attack, but it was soon overshadowed by fear and guilt. What could I possibly say to my parents when they found out about it in the morning?

When they did find out the next day, all I could think of to do was plead ignorance. I told them that I didn't know what happened, and I couldn't explain it. My parents must have known that I was responsible, but they did not accuse me or blame me. I think that they probably discussed it with each other, but they never brought it up with me.

The lie that I told then now seems inevitable under the circumstances, but in the end, I don't think that it served me or my family well. They were not, nor was I, able to face and deal with the open expression of our own anger. It was just too frightening.

Around the same age I had another challenging emotional experience. I used to walk back and forth to school with a girl who lived in my building. The walk took us through a park in a rough neighborhood.

One day on our way home, I was lagging behind her, and I was accosted by a group of three or four boys, while she had not been stopped, and she walked on ahead. These boys were proteges of street gangs, who were known as the *bishops'* and the *chaplains*. As pre-teens they were called *baby bishops* and *baby chaplains*. They pushed me around a little and punched me a few times. Seeing my dark, curly hair, the ringleader asked, "Are you Italian? Cause I'm a spic (Puerto Rican), and I don't like no Italians!"

"No, no. I'm Jewish!" I pleaded. My physical injuries were minimal, but I was very scared. My female friend had seen it all, from a safe distance. When I caught up with her, I didn't want her to see me cry, but there was no way I could prevent it. I cried, and she said it would be OK. She comforted me. It felt humiliating to cry in front of a girl, and to let her comfort me. I was glad that there was no one else around.

P.S. 117—junior high school

I continued to live in Kingsview and to go to the local public school, Francis Scott Key Junior High. Once again, I was happy to be put on the fast track, or "special progress" (S.P.) class, which meant that students would cover the educational material for seventh, eighth, and ninth grades in two years.

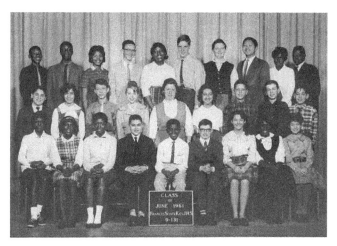

My ninth-grade class. I am in the back row, fourth from the left.

I continued to stand out academically in junior high. I was editor-in-chief of *ScottLite*, which was a combined yearbook and literary magazine. There was even a valedictorian in junior high school, and it was I. Three years later I was to be valedictorian at Stuyvesant High School.

It was in junior high that I first experienced anti-Semitism firsthand, which felt personal and painful. One girl in my class and I felt a mutual, early adolescent, romantic attraction. She would sometimes go home with me after school to my apartment in Kingsview. Our excuse to ourselves (which she initiated), and to any others who might care, was that she needed to "look up something in the *Encyclopedia Britannica*," which my parents had bought for Les and me, and which had no equivalent in her house. (This was long before the Internet and Google.)

My brother was off at college, and my parents were at work, so she and I were home alone for an hour or two. As I recall, we might have looked something up in the encyclopedia once or twice, but mostly we just fooled around and got excited. She was a blond, blue-eyed Dutch-American girl. When her father found out about us, she told me that her father said he didn't want her to be going out with *a Jew-boy*! That ended our relationship. I was never able to talk about it or process that incident with my parents or anyone else. As I recall, I even feared at one point that it was she who wanted to end our romance, such as it was, and since she seemed good at inventing excuses, she might have used her father (whom I never met) as an excuse for ending it.

I had one teacher in junior high who I really liked. Fred Khoury was my social studies teacher for both of the years I was there. He was the only teacher whom my parents ever invited to dinner at our apartment. That was special. But there is also an embarrassing part to this. Sometimes well-intentioned white people like my father tried to gain favor with people of color by impressing them with how much *we* know about *their* culture. As I remember it, my father cooked a leg of lamb for dinner, and he told Mr. Khoury that he understood *you people* like lamb, *and* that you like it cooked rare. (Mr. Khoury was an Arab.) I felt mortified at the time.

The embarrassment which I felt about my father's unaware anti-Arab racism did not translate for me into embarrassment about the same sort of racism which I displayed, without much awareness, mostly toward African Heritage people. Until very recently, I would still try to impress black folks, by showing them how much I knew about *their* (presumed) history or culture. Or I might do something that was not characteristic for me, like giving a black man a *high five*. Given the racist conditioning that we all grew up with, it makes sense that I still have some work to do to become an effective ally to people of color (whom I now refer to as people of the *global* majority/indigenous or PGMI.)

Summer of '62 at Howard University

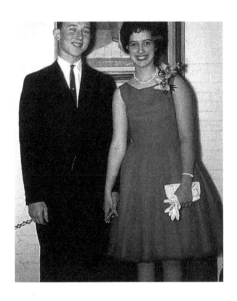

In the summer of 1962, I was fourteen years old and had just finished my first year of high school. The civil rights movement had started to make the nightly news. In the South, with the likes of Police Chief "Bull" Connor, and of Alabama Governor George Wallace, who vowed, "segregation now, segregation forever." John Lewis and Dr. Martin Luther King, Jr. were young non-violent idealists confronting *the system*. To me, it was an exciting time, but the violence was also scary to me. I had never lived away from home, even to go to summer camp.

My parents found a summer program for me, hoping to give my science education at Stuyvesant a boost. It was sponsored by the National Science Foundation. There I could take a few courses and work alongside a mentor at a university on a science research project. I didn't have a lot of work to do, and I had time to pursue other fun things, such as glass blowing, seeing the sights, and meeting girls.

My parents thought that it was an extra benefit that the program which they chose for me was at Howard University, in Washington, DC. This, they thought, could advance my understanding of racism and progressive politics up close. They explained to me that Howard was one of a number of tradition-ally black colleges. There was a lot of sightseeing to do in Washington, DC, and although it was the seat of the federal government, it also had the feel of a Southern city.

Apparently, the program's plan was for white stu-dents from the North and black students from the South to meet each other, to learn and understand each other. This plan was only partially successful. In the cafeteria and elsewhere, we pretty much self-seg-regated. And racism had already infected us by that age. It didn't help that some white male students got physically attacked by black teenagers (although they were not from the program) early on in the summer. Over most of my life, I have felt more comfortable around women, of any color, than with men, of any color, because of the social conditioning of people by gender, as well by race. I got to know a couple of black girls at Howard, but not well, and I went gallivanting around town with a couple of white girls. We visited the Washington and Lincoln Memorials, the National Cathedral, a synagogue, and an A.M.E. Church (with one of the black girls). One of the white girls became my first real love.

She was from Philadelphia and went to an all-girls public high school. I was from New York and went to an all-boys public high school. We also discovered that we shared the *red diaper* identity. Both of us were children of parents on the far left. Neither of us was old enough to drive. My parents had driven me down to DC, and they were planning to bring me home by car as well. I asked them whether they could bring my girlfriend back to her home in Philly at the end of the summer since it was not too far out of our way; otherwise, she would have had to take the Amtrak train home. They agreed, and so our parents met also. She and I wrote letters back and forth that fall, and she invited me to her junior prom. So my parents drove me back and forth between New York and Philadelphia. I remember showing up at her door carrying a corsage for her to wear at the prom.

But alas, it was just a summer love, too difficult to sustain across time and distance. She and I
lost touch with each other until very recently. We
did then tell each other our stories of how our lives
had gone since that summer of 1962, and we both
found it very interesting, but the narrative of the
two of us pretty much ends after the junior prom.

Stuyvesant High School

In some large cities in the US, the public school system includes specialized high schools, often requiring an entrance exam in ninth grade. In New York at that time there were three special science schools—Brooklyn Technical HS, Stuyvesant HS, and the Bronx High School of Science. The same entrance exam was required for all of them, but students were allowed to choose which one they attended.

I lived quite close to Brooklyn Tech, but I chose not to go there, probably out of snobbery based on the idea that it focused more on technical trades, rather than on pure science, but also because my brother had gone to Stuyvesant, graduating as valedictorian just before I enrolled. Bronx Science was widely thought to be the best of the three and was known throughout the US, but the long commute took it out of consideration for me.

The High School of Music and Art was also a NYC public school, which required an entrance exam and an audition, I believe. It was also in Manhattan, but that school never even appeared on my radar. A smart Jewish boy should go into science, medicine, or law, not art. Besides, my artistic skills to that point were only in classical ballet, and

I'm not sure that Music and Art even had a dance program, although I didn't try to find out.

I entered Stuyvesant in the fall of 1961, and I graduated in 1964 as valedictorian. Approximately 75 percent of the students were Jews, who were part of the *upwardly mobile* trend of second- and third-generation Jewish Americans at that time. (In recent years, the majority of the student body has been Asian. Asians now represent the bulk of the group who have recently immigrated to US cities, and they are now *upwardly mobile*. And Stuyvesant is now co-ed instead of all boys, which might give it a chance to catch up to Bronx Science, which was co-ed from the beginning). Unlike my elementary school and my junior high, blacks were a small minority, and there were very few Puerto Ricans.

One unfortunate result of being an all-boys school was the absence of girls! This meant that we boys were able to continue to assume that girls were inferior academically; more importantly, we weren't able to socialize easily with them. I think that Stuyvesant had a *sister school*, Hunter College high school, but I don't remember any social events, or *mixers* with them. Somehow, in junior and senior years I met a lovely girl who went to the High School of Music and Art. There was very little touching, and certainly no sex. One other Stuyvesant boy was my rival for her affections. The most wonderful memory I have from that time was a concert that the three of us went to, on Christmas Eve at midnight, at Carnegie Hall. The entire oratorio of Handel's Messiah was played, with an orchestra and chorus. When the Hallelujah chorus was played, the entire sold-out audience got to our feet and sang along. ("And he shall live forever and ever...") Another eye-opening experience for this secular Jew!

Organized sports were not emphasized at Stuyvesant, but we won a few games in a few sports (the chess, debating, and math teams always did very well). Two of my good friends, Ted Gold and Ric Quinones ran track. Ric (possibly the only Puerto Rican in my class of eight hundred) was very fast in sprints. Ric knew from gym class that I was good at standing broad jump, so he invited me to join the team in the spring of our senior year, to do running long jump and triple jump. Why not? We knew that we could win by forfeit if the other team had no one to compete in those events. I did win a few meets by forfeit, but I also managed to medal in a few meets as well.

In spring of 1964 we graduated, and Ted went off to Columbia. I got into Harvard, as did Ric.

We both felt pleased and a little intimidated, as two kids from Brooklyn who were about to enter a very prestigious college before we turned seventeen. Ric and I decided to be freshman roommates.

Teddy deserves a chapter of his own in my story.

Ted Gold

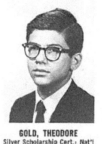

GOLD, THEODORE
Silver Scholarship Cert.; Nat'l
Merit Commendation; Bronze
PSAL Award; Track & Cross-
Country Teams; Forum Staff;
Stamp Club; History & Folk-
lore Soc.

*For someone who
spent 3(3) years
in this place you
didn't turn out
too bad. Ted*

I first met Ted Gold in the fall of 1961, when we entered Stuyvesant in the tenth grade, at the age of fourteen. We graduated in June 1964.

The civil rights movement had been in full swing for a few years at that point. We watched on TV, as non-violent protestors, most of them black but some white, got clubbed and tear-gassed, and were pushed back by high-pressure water hoses. The Student Non-Violent Coordinating Committee (SNCC) was active in the South, and they became our heroes. We formed the High School Friends of SNCC, which for us morphed into SDS, after 1964.

The war in Vietnam was also heating up as well, and we formed Lower Manhattan Students for Peace. Ted and I both came from progressive Jewish families, who fought to make the world better and more just. Although we didn't see each other outside of school much when we were at Stuyvesant, I visited him at home a few times, where he lived with his parents, Hy and Ruth. We also shared some cynicism about our school principal and many other adults.

Ted was willing to push the boundaries of insolence at times, while I always felt more cautious. I was a more serious student, and more serious in general. Essentially, I think that I was more scared than Teddy. I wanted to keep my high academic standing. I had a model to follow in my older brother. Ted had a younger brother. Les had been the valedictorian at Stuyvesant in 1960, and he went on from there to Harvard, on full scholarship. Not to be outdone, I was the valedictorian in 1964 and went on to Harvard on full scholarship as well.

Ted had also done well academically in high school, and he went to Columbia College. We continued to share our affection for each other. In my high school yearbook, Ted wrote, "For someone who spent 3(3) years in this place, you didn't turn out too bad" The 3(3) reference was a goofy ref-

erence to the frequent redundancies which seemed
to turn up sometimes on our exam instructions.
We stayed committed to each other and to social
change. We were both active in SDS, but we stayed
only loosely connected to each other during those
years. At some point in high school, he gave me
a little printed card about air-raid drills in school,
which read:

"What to do in the event of nuclear attack:

1. Hide under your desk.
2. Put your head between your knees.
3. Kiss your ass good-bye!"

I kept that card in my wallet for years.

It was frustrating to us protestors that the US
pursued the war in Vietnam both vigorously and
viciously. The Vietnamese were mostly rural peas-
ants, yet they fought heroically against a super-
power. All sorts of terrible things were happening
there.

The US army troops referred to the Vietnamese
people as *gooks*. US troops were being worn down by
the irregular army known as the Viet Cong. Feeling
mutinous, some of the US army *grunts* actually
killed their commanding officers by *fragging* them,
using fragmentation grenades. It was entirely cha-

otic, and the abbreviation PTSD came into common usage at that time.

We left-wing students felt impotent and frustrated politically. We couldn't stop the war. What started as protracted debates over tactics in our political groups developed into opposing factions, each insisting that their ideas were the *correct line*. We learned later that the FBI had agents who infiltrated SDS and gave SDS a little push toward its inevitable splintering in 1968. Three factions resulted. The most adventurist, impatient, and violent were the Weathermen. "You don't need a Weatherman to know which way the wind blows" (Bob Dylan).

The Weathermen actually believed that *the Revolution* was imminent. They decided that they would work together with the Black Panther Party to make this happen. SDS had come a long way in a short time, from the Student Non-Violent Coordinating Committee to a group embracing violence to promote social change.

Ted and I had kept in touch through our college years, but our views diverged. None of the three former SDS factions seemed attractive to me. After graduating from Harvard in 1968 and moving back to New York, I helped form the short-lived and very local Movement for a Democratic Society. Teddy became a Weatherman. I never saw him again.

On March 6, 1971, he died in a massive explosion that destroyed a townhouse on Eleventh Street in Manhattan, when a bomb that his *cell* was making detonated prematurely in the basement, killing Ted and two others. Two others survived.

Ellen and I were living on Thirteenth Street at the time, and Ted must have made the others aware that I lived nearby, and that I was loyal to him personally, even though we didn't agree politically. I had already known many people from SDS before they joined the Weathermen. The two survivors appeared at my door as soon as they could flee from the destroyed townhouse. One had wounds which needed to be dressed. They didn't stay very long at my place. Within a couple of hours, they went off to places unknown. They were now fugitives from the law. They became part of the group which they renamed the Weather Underground, and they managed to evade capture for many months.

At this point, I am able to think about all this more dispassionately. We were twenty-two years old. I was terribly sad but also very angry at Ted for making this huge political error, which was ultimately self-destructive. I did consider our personality differences, but this time I didn't feel bad about being more timid and less rebellious than he was—

this time I thought that caution served me well. I was more level-headed; he was more hot-headed.

I was closer to my working-class roots, so maybe I was able to take a longer view of the pace of social transformation. I was the first doctor in my family. I grew up in a tough neighborhood in Brooklyn. I didn't believe that *the Revolution* was imminent. I had started out in life in a small house, living with my parents and grandparents.

Ted's father was himself a doctor and a liberal Jew, and Ted grew up with his parents, living in a high-rise apartment building on the Upper East Side of Manhattan. Most of the leadership of the Weathermen, as far as I could tell, were well-educated white people from middle or owning class backgrounds. The townhouse on Eleventh Street belonged to the parents of one of the survivors, and the other was the daughter of a prominent defense attorney. My belief is that these young peoples' judgment was clouded, mostly by impatience. They wanted so much to make the world right, and they thought, unrealistically, that they should be able to make the revolution happen very soon.

I still grieve for Ted Gold.

Shall I dance?

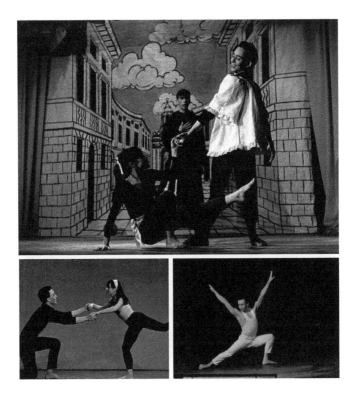

I loved dancing, and I was good at it. I started in ballet at age eleven, somewhat arbitrarily, when Mrs. Farrar agreed to do a favor for the older sister of a boy in our class. She *volunteered* three of us boys to go to an all-boys class at her dancing school. My liberal parents did not object. I loved it. It wasn't very long before I started *partnering* ballerinas. I became their young *premier danseur*. I loved watching the New York City Ballet and other professional dance companies. I was totally enthralled by movies of musical theater, especially "West Side Story." I pursued my dance studies, but I kept it quiet during my years in an all-boys high school.

Actually, for my English honors' project as a senior at Stuyvesant, I wrote a thirty-page paper (with footnotes), titled "Men in Ballet?" This was an apologia to explain and justify myself. I used some great titles for book references (which had only limited relevance to the topic), such as "The Dance of Life" by Havelock Ellis. My father had always approved of my dancing (in part, no doubt, due to his own limitations after his foot was amputated as a young man). He fed me the first line for my paper: "Man has always been a dancer."

I thought that I was probably good enough to dance professionally, although I also knew that it was not an easy way to make a living. My father's advice about what to do when I grew up had two criteria: (1) do something that you're good at, and (2) do something that the world needs. I would say at *this* point in my life that the world needs dance and art and beauty. But when I was sixteen, and very serious, this was less clear to me. It seemed clearer to me that pursuing a career in science would be helpful to the world. And there was still the issue of actually being able to make a decent living as a performer. And finally, I was a confirmed heterosexual, having absorbed the homophobia which was largely unchallenged at the time. It is true in our culture that many classical male dancers are gay, and that was off-putting to me. One of my heroes was a male dancer in the NYC Ballet who was married to a female dancer, and she kept on performing past the time that her pregnancy obviously showed.

As a last hurrah for me, or as an attempt to get the urge to perform out of my system, I went away to summer camp at age sixteen for the first time in my life. It was the summer before I was headed to Harvard to study Biology. The camp was on Cape Cod, and it was called Dartmuthe, an acronym for dance, art, music, and theater. At camp that summer, I got to dance, and not only ballet. I got to sing and act a little too. All the departments were open to all the students. The dance department consisted of two men, who were both gay. As dance teachers, I thought that they were just adequate. And of course, they never *came on* to me in any way. I can tell by my reactions to them all these years later that I still have some work to do before I'm really able to let go of my homophobia.

Well, that summer didn't dissuade me in the least from my love of dance nor the enjoyment I took in performing. I found a way to continue dancing when I got to Harvard. During my freshman year at Harvard, I saw a poster inviting dancers to join the Harvard-Radcliffe Jazz Dance Workshop. They welcomed men who were actually trained dancers; I joined, and I loved it. The first year that I was there, a Harvard senior directed. The next year, a classmate of mine directed. And in the final year, I directed. (No women directed during the time that I was there.) It was well run, with people helping with advertising, tech, scenery, photography, etc. I danced in many of the numbers, and I choreographed some, too. I did one solo piece for myself, set to a sermon poem, "The Creation," by James Weldon Johnson. The poem was read, offstage, by one of my SDS roommates who had a strong bass voice. One of the dances, early on, which I did not choreograph myself, turned out to be a turning point for me in the trajectory of my life!

In this dance, I played the part of an altar boy(!) in Italy at the time of the *commedia dell'arte* and I was fascinated by the *cantatrice* from the troupe. We did a duet which was just beautiful. Indeed, we fell in love offstage as well, and I married Ellen just after my Harvard graduation, when I was not yet twenty-one years old. We took off to Europe for a summer honeymoon on a shoestring budget, between college and medical school. We were able to stay together through my medical school years, but our marriage did not survive 1973, which was a stressful internship year for me, and a time of extreme turmoil in our country and the rest of the world.

Freshmen at Harvard—Ric and I

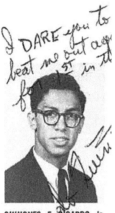

I DARE you to beat me out aga-
st in th
for

QUINONES, E. RICARDO, Jr.
Arista; Jr. Arista; Gold
Scholarship Cert.; Nat'l Merit
Semi-Finalist; Spanish Cert.;
Gold PSAL Award; Off. Cl.
; Pres. & Vice-Pres.; Capt.
Track Team; Cross Country
Team; Spectator Staff; Library
Squad.

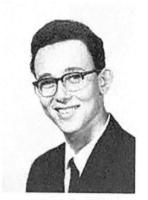

LESSINGER, ERIC
Arista; Gold Scholarship Cert.;
Nat'l Merit Semi-finalist;
French Cert.; Silver PSAL
Award; Off. Cl. Pres.; Pres.
Bio-Med Soc.; Band; Biology
Tutor.

My parents drove me from Brooklyn to Cambridge and helped get me settled in Pennypacker Hall, one of the freshman dorms. I had a few items I brought with me. My parents stayed overnight, and they left the next day. I was in a double room with Ric Quinones, my high school classmate. Ric's presence helped me feel less disoriented, as did the presence of my older brother Les, who had just graduated but who was in graduate school right there at Harvard. The whole scene was very new, and the physical setting and the social culture took some getting used to.

Soon Ric and I got busy with coursework. We also scanned the Radcliffe freshman register, to try and see who the *Cliffies* were, where their home towns were, and whether we could recognize any of the ones who were in our incoming class from their pictures, when we saw them in classes or out and about. At that time, Radcliffe was still a separate college, but all of our classes were together.

Ric and I didn't socialize with each other much. We soon fell in with different crowds. My political beliefs were very important to me: I was on the far left, and I became increasingly active, demonstrating against the war in Vietnam, etc. My parents mostly approved. Ric and his parents were liberal, but his family may have kept their distance from politics during those years. We started together at Harvard in the fall of 1964, and we graduated in the spring of 1968.

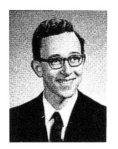

ERIC LESSINGER
Born on January 31, 1948 at Brooklyn, New York. Prepared at Stuyvesant High School, New York, New York. Home Address: 105 Ashland Place, Brooklyn, New York. Field of Concentration: Biology. Phillips Brooks House Association; Students for a Democratic Society, Chairman 65; Jazz Dance Workshop. Harvard College Scholarship; National Honor Society Scholarship.

My Harvard College '68 yearbook
photo with accompanying bio.

Les and I at Harvard

I am very grateful to Les for all the advice he gave me as I navigated my way through Harvard. He and Hanna stayed on at Harvard as graduate students, so they lived nearby in Cambridge. Les advised me to take the well-known survey courses Fine Arts 13 and Music 1. I knew that I wanted to study science but rather than start out with upper-level courses for which I could qualify, Les recommended that I take Natural Sciences 5, an introductory-level Biology course taught by George Wald, who in addition to being a Nobel Prize winner, was also a very good teacher and a kindly man.

Harvard had a *house* system for student living. When I moved to the *off-campus house*, which wasn't really a physical house at all, I continued to live with my SDS comrades. Les and Hanna continued to provide good support for me, and I was able to meet other people through them and to see my own friends in the privacy of their apartment.

I finally broke away from Les's path when he stayed at Harvard to complete his PhD in Physical Chemistry, and I went to New York University Medical School in July 1968.

My years at Harvard

Early on in freshman year, my path diverged from Ric's. We were both smart working-class kids from Brooklyn whose families wanted us very much for us to succeed. My dad was an accountant; his dad was a postal worker.

We both looked at the Radcliffe freshman register and saw the pictures and read the profiles of the *Cliffies*. There were a few Jews among them, judging by their names, and probably no Puerto Ricans, but a few Latinas. Some in their class, comprising three hundred or so, lived outside of the US, and many went to private schools which I had never heard of. (The same was true for our Harvard class of one thousand two hundred or so). Finding a young woman to communicate with was a challenge, in the absence of email and private phones. We recognized a few of them from their pictures, walking across the quad. I don't remember going to any parties, or *mixers* at all. I certainly felt more than a little intimidated. I might have gone on one date with a Radcliffe student during my entire time at Harvard.

Ric started hanging out and going to parties with a different crowd, who drank, and may have had connections with women, possibly with women from Radcliffe, or possibly with one of the nearby women's colleges. There were also *parietal rules* for us, which included curfews for visits. Dorm room doors needed to be open *at least the width of a book*, and couples were required to have at least one foot on the floor at all times. (Seriously!)

The war in Vietnam was heating up, and I got right into the thick of the protest movement at Harvard. The largest protest group was the Students for a Democratic Society (SDS). There were a dozen or more freshmen from Harvard and Radcliffe ready to join, in 1964. We held lots of meetings, to discuss political positions, strategies, and tactics, and to plan some demonstrations. Seven of us decided to room together in Adams House, in an adjoining triple and a quad. We remain friends to this day. (Except for Hal Benenson, who committed suicide after his wife died of breast cancer at age twenty-nine). I was chosen to be Chairman of Harvard-Radcliffe SDS for 1965–1966.

That was also the year when Robert McNamara came to speak at the Kennedy School of Government to a select group of graduate students and faculty. (McNamara was Secretary of Defense for LBJ.) We were fired up and ready. "Hey, hey, LBJ, how many kids did you kill today?" "Murderer!"

The Secret Service and Cambridge Police knew that we planned to demonstrate. When McNamara was ready to leave Harvard, they sent out a decoy car, as well as the limo with him in it. We got wind of it and rushed over to his car. My brother Les was one of the students who sat down in front of the car, preventing McNamara from driving off. The Cambridge Police were in full riot gear, with helmets, batons, and plastic shields. They slowly pushed us back, but not before we were able to get McNamara to get out and address the crowd. He was obviously angry and flustered, with a beefy-red face. He spoke of his younger days, memorably saying, "I was tougher than you then, and I'm tougher than you now!" Eventually he left, but we counted it as a victory for our side.

Soon thereafter, Dean Ford, the dean of students, called me into his office, asking for an explanation. I said something like, "Well, I guess that some of my members got a little too enthusiastic." He was not pleased. The one hundred or so of us whom they could identify were put on probation. I do remember a demonstration later when we held up signs which read, "On pro, and proud of it!" Those were heady and contentious times. We thought we were on the verge of massive social change.

Academically I continued to do well. My lowest grade was a C, in Organic Chemistry, a pre-med prerequisite. I graduated cum laude in 1968. Then on to medical school!

Section 3: **MEDICAL TRAINING**

Preparing for med school

I do take credit for making two decisions based on my best *thinking*, rather than my *feelings*, as I got ready to enter medical school. The first was about the military draft. The war in Vietnam did not affect all young people in the US equally. There was no volunteer army. Young men who were poor, be they black, brown, or white, were being drafted into the army and were being shipped off to fight and die in Vietnam. Young men were sorted into classifications before being drafted. If you passed a pre-induction physical exam at your local draft board, you would then be classified 1-A, meaning you were physically fit to serve if drafted, or, if you were physically unfit, you would be classified 4-F. The doctor for Donald J. Trump found *bone spurs* in him, to do this legal bit of draft dodging.

There was also a separate category for the psychologically or morally unfit. You can get the flavor of it by listening to Arlo Guthrie singing "Alice's Restaurant." And then, for full-time students, there was the possibility of deferring military service until after you had completed your education. The student deferment gave you a classification of 2-S. I had a student deferment at Harvard, but I did not re-apply for it in the summer of 1968, before I started medical school. I thought it was only fair to take my chances with the war machine like other young men. And a game of chance it was.

There was a draft *lottery*, so that all of us would be chosen based on our birthdays, which were randomly assigned to a number from 1 to 365. Number 1 would be the first to get called up, and so on. My number was over 300. I got *lucky*, but I was glad that I made the decision nonetheless. I didn't get called up. The tremendously unpopular war led to a lot of changes, including the end of the draft, and ultimately to the US pulling out of the war, but not winning the war. That war had no truce and no winner.

The second good decision I made was to learn more about the working people whose daily jobs as janitors or nurses' aides allowed the medical system to function, before I took my place at the top of the medical hierarchy.

As an *upwardly mobile* Jewish man I decided that I wanted to be a doctor. I used the summer between my Harvard graduation and my NYU enrollment to work as an aide at a nursing home. I was twenty years old, and I had essentially no work experience. Most of the aides were women of color, but I was assigned to a considerably older white man to be my mentor at the nursing home. He taught me how to position bedpans and how to empty them safely and cleanly; how to change bed linens, including making hospital corners, a lot about how to handle patients, rolling patients on their sides to change the sheets for patients who could not get out of bed; safe transfers from bed to chair and back; and more. It was humbling and enlightening. It was clearly not a job that I wanted to do long term. I joined my classmates later that summer secure in the knowledge that I had learned something important. Doing working-class jobs could bring people closer to their co-workers and to the people in their care. Also that being a hospital aide was not a job that I wanted to do on a full-time permanent basis.

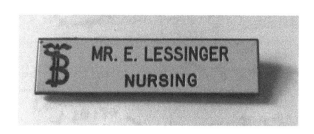

Medical school begins

Recently married, Ellen and I moved to an apartment on East Thirteenth Street in Manhattan. Ellen found work as an administrative assistant at a neighborhood health center called NENA (the North East Neighborhood Association of the Lower East Side), and there she made good connections with the doctors and social workers, as well as their families. Several years later, after we divorced, she became a doctor herself.

It was only two short stops north on the subway from our apartment to the medical school. Depending on how much time it took to walk to school or to wait for the next train, and depending upon the weather outside, I could get to First Avenue and Thirtieth Street in just about the same period of time either way. I arrived at NYU Medical School in the early fall of 1968.

The first week or two were a blur. There were one hundred and forty or so classmates to meet. Probably fifty or so were Jewish. The only classmate I knew when I got there was my SDS roommate from Harvard. There were fifteen or so women in the class (that demographic has changed; women are now 50 percent or more of medical students.) I had only one black classmate. The medical school was housed in a single building, with classrooms, teaching labs, and a student lounge. As I remember it, gross anatomy (dissecting cadavers) was in the windowless basement. It all seemed to be coming at me too quickly.

University Hospital was a *private* hospital, also in one building, but it was a huge looming tower just across the street from the medical school. Most of our training actually took place at Bellevue Hospital, which was a *public hospital*, run by a New York City agency. It was even bigger than University Hospital, and although its name had become synonymous with a *lunatic asylum* it actually was a full-service hospital. The third hospital in the NYU system was the Manhattan VA Hospital, run by the Veteran's Agency, a federal department.

As I mentioned earlier, NYU displayed a lot less snobbery than Harvard. There were few, if any, students who had grown up owning class. There were no *legacy admissions*, as there were at Harvard. There was no unstated quota on Jews at NYU, as I am sure there had been at Harvard College.

Skipping ahead in this story to the yearbook published when we finished our time there, class of 1972, I am struck by several things. What strikes me first is the fashion of young people between 1968 and 1972. Lots of long hair and facial hair.

And our class had lots of married couples; some of them both doctors. Smoking was still socially acceptable; many male students (as well as faculty) were pictured smoking cigars, pipes, and cigarettes, trying to look sophisticated, or at least pleased with themselves.

I looked very young. (I was twenty-four when I graduated). I was also struck, in retrospect, by the warm camaraderie which I felt for almost half the class, partly because many of us shared progressive politics in those days, and partly because we had been through some difficult times together during training.

The first year

And so, the fun began. At first, our experience was confined almost completely to the classroom. For the first two years we studied basic medical sciences—physiology, anatomy, neuroanatomy, biochemistry, pharmacology, genetics, microbiology, hematology. We did get to go to the hospital for *clinical correlation* (usually to Bellevue, where the attending physicians had no *private patients*); there the clinical faculty could demonstrate physical findings on live human subjects.

Our only other introduction to the human body in the first year was our cadaver. Four of us would gather around a steel table, spending many hours carefully dissecting an embalmed body. Some groups actually named their cadavers, which was partly an attempt to humanize them, and partly to make light of the situation in order to defend themselves against feeling its ghastliness. As I recall, I did find it somewhat humorous, although at my table we didn't give our cadaver a name.

The whole scene in those years encouraged callousness. There was no group processing. There was no emotional support at the school. Maybe at home, there was someone who could listen. The psychiatry department was there to teach us about patients' psychopathology, not to help us deal with the depression or anxiety which was common among medical students. Fortunately, as far as I know, there was no suicide at NYU during the time I was there (unlike at Harvard), despite the intense pressure of our training. There was a student health service, where we were all given physical exams upon entry to the school. Many of us never went back there again. There were no general practitioners on the faculty, so there was not likely to be an avuncular mentor who might remind me of my own GP when I was growing up.

We were being trained to be at the top of the social and professional hierarchy—mostly representing respected, wealthy, white, US-born males. As such, it was easy to slip into arrogance, and into the assumption that we were better and smarter than everybody else. Some items in our 1972 yearbook seemed genuinely funny, but it's embarrassing to me now to read the book, which was written by my classmates. It oozes pomposity, sophomoric humor, and disrespect. I was struck by some quotes in the yearbook which contained words spoken by a faculty member whose English was heavily accented. These words were spelled out phonetically, which made them sound *funny*. I cringe at the thought that this faculty member might have read it. I would have felt insulted.

¡Venceremos!

Between the first and second years of medical school, I hoped to work as a volunteer in Cuba. In 1959, Fidel Castro's army overthrew the dictator Fulgencio Batista, becoming the first communist regime established in my lifetime, as well as the first communist regime in the Western Hemisphere. The US government was quite hostile. There was fear-mongering (after all, Cuba was just ninety miles from Miami!). An embargo on sales between the US and Cuba was instituted, as was a travel ban. Our government organized and financed a small army to invade Cuba by boat at Playa Giron (the Bay of Pigs). It was a miserable failure, and the US government initially denied that it was involved. Most galling of all, the US owned a small piece of land which should have been part of Cuba: the US Naval Base at Guantanamo Bay. This facility was used as a prison, and it gained notoriety for its cruel torture techniques, including *water-boarding*, which was against international law.

The prospect of being part of a revolutionary society was exciting to me. The first Venceremos Brigade traveled in the winter. But I was a full-time student, as were many other young people who wanted to go. Therefore it was decided that the second brigade would travel over the course of the next summer, to accommodate students' schedules. My application to the brigade was accepted, and I met with other accepted participants regularly, to be vetted by the program, to get to know the other participants somewhat and to practice some Spanish language.

Unfortunately, the calendar at NYU Medical School required me to start earlier than many other colleges or graduate schools by three weeks or so. This didn't seem to me to be an obstacle which could not be overcome. I thought that I could skip the first six-week unit, and then make it up, probably by extending my year into the next summer.

I decided to explain my plan to the school. I made an appointment with the dean of students to discuss it. Once he realized the purpose of my absence, he said, "You can go to Cuba, but if you do, don't expect to come back to this school." That ended my hopes of going to Cuba with the brigade. I feared that I would be risking my career, and I was not willing to do that. I stayed in school, and I didn't go on the Venceremos Brigade.

Choosing not to go to Cuba seemed rational. It was a bigger risk than I was willing to take. I did what the school and society expected of me. Later, I wondered what would have happened if I had simply showed up late, without prior notice. In retrospect, asking for permission, and thereby giving notice to the powers-that-be, might have been another option. I was too scared even to imagine taking the risk.

The second year

During the second year, in addition to doing course work, we inched closer to clinical work. Each of us was assigned to a single patient at Bellevue to perform a complete history and physical exam. A small group of us were assigned to follow one faculty member around like a group of ducklings. Then each of us in turn had to give a presentation of the patient assigned to us, in front of a small group of our peers. We all stood around the bedside and presented *the case*. We presented the history and demonstrated the physical findings on the patients' body right there.

Sometimes our mentor would demonstrate a technique, or ask one of the others to demonstrate a technique, such as percussing the lungs or liver. The patient, who was right there, was only occasionally asked a question or communicated with in any way. Sometimes the patient only spoke Spanish, which we students were not expected to learn. In that case, there were references sometimes made to *veterinary medicine*. I don't recall feeling humiliated in the process myself, but sometimes it felt almost as painful when I was watching it happen to one of my classmates.

At the completion of the second year, we took the first part of the exam administered by the National Board of Medical Examiners. I think we all passed the exam, and then it was on to the third and fourth years, when, after a few more hurdles, we would train to be MDs!

The third year

The third year was a reprise of the clinical part of the second year. In the third year we left the classrooms and spent all of our time in the hospital, seeing patients, making teaching rounds, and visiting the library. The physical exams (H&Ps) were now done on a whole small panel of patients which we were each assigned to. We then had to present the patient (*the case*) verbally to an attending physician (*attending*).

Going down the hierarchy, there was a chief resident, who covered the entire panel of either medical or surgical or pediatric patients, with first and second-year residents who reported to them, and then came the intern, who at least had an MD after his or her name, and finally us, the students. The attendings were paid a salary for teaching at Bellevue or the Manhattan VA Hospital. It was only at University Hospital that the attendings had their private patients, who probably had to agree to be seen by doctors-in-training as a condition of their hospitalization, but their experience was definitely different. They appeared to be comfortable and knowledgeable, were treated with respect, and participated in their own history and physical exam.

They all spoke English, and occasionally joked with their *real doctor.*

For us to report the patient's story to the attending physician, and to tell them what we found on their physical exam (*presenting the case*) was intentionally intimidating. Some of the faculty were kind, but the culture and traditions of medicine were generally designed to toughen us up emotionally and to learn how to work despite sleep deprivation. It was not OK to be unprepared in any way, or to make a mistake. It was a setup for humiliation in front of our peers. If I couldn't answer the doctor's question, then he'd see if there was anyone else who could. And if a student couldn't answer, then the intern or resident had better know the answer! Usually all this took place at the bedside, in front of the patient. Occasionally the attending doctor would ask the patient an important question which we had failed to ask, or he/she would point out a physical finding which we had missed.

This didn't usually inspire confidence in us from our patients. We knew that we were not doctors yet, and of course, we didn't feel confident. We hoped that our patients would not find out about any mistakes that we might have made. On the other hand, we were not yet doctors, and so we were closer to the patients in that way, and sometimes we had moments of genuine, gratifying human interaction. Likewise, when we were not competing with our classmates, we could commiserate with each other, debrief, and tell stories.

The classes in basic medical sciences of the first two years gave way to clinical rotations in the third year, which were mandatory periods of six weeks each in the hospital to learn about internal medicine, pediatrics, surgery, and shorter periods to study radiology and anesthesia. While on the longer rotations, we had to be available at all hours, so we slept in the hospital, in *on-call* rooms.

It seemed to me that surgical on-call was the most challenging. The practice of surgery itself could be very gratifying to the surgeon and the patient, but its appeal to me was limited because what I saw of it in the hospital allowed little time for interaction. I suppose that more interesting discussions were happening in the office, before surgery. Come to think of it, there was no requirement for *any* outpatient training in any field that I can recall, and most of us wouldn't have thought of taking six weeks of entirely outpatient training as an elective period.

The third year was probably the most difficult one for most of us.

The fourth year

In the fourth and final year (for most of us, with the exception of the *mud-fuds* who went for six years usually, to come out with an MD as well as a PhD in a related field), things eased up a bit. We still had some prescribed clinical rotations, but we could set up elective rotations as well, such as public health or rehabilitation medicine, sometimes in New York, but sometimes elsewhere in the US or abroad. These were life-changing experiences for many of us. I arranged for a *sub-internship* at Ganado, Arizona, on the Navajo Indian Reservation, for the winter of 1971–1972.

On the Navajo reservation

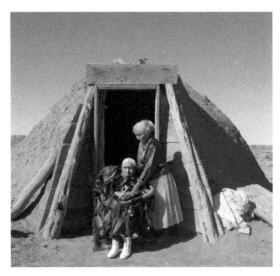

Navajo women in front of their hogan.

Project Hope was a humanitarian organization which had projects worldwide, including medical aid to the Navajo Nation on its large reservation in Arizona. It was the winter of 1971–1972 when I arrived at the village of Ganado, Arizona.

I worked there for two months as a *sub-intern*, that is, I was not yet an MD, but I would be going into my internship year after graduating from medical school. I worked at Sage Memorial Hospital, which had been established years earlier as part of a Presbyterian mission, and whose small, all-white medical staff still had a Christian missionary feel to it. The staff were self-sacrificing, they didn't allow themselves to feel much, and they seemed distant from their (Navajo and Hopi) patients. This whole scene made me uncomfortable, as a Jewish kid from Brooklyn.

Sage Memorial was a twenty-five-bed facility, and I was under the supervision of an experienced general practitioner, who was well trained, and who cared about his patients. My work schedule was every day shift (twelve hours). Also alternating night shifts on call (twelve hours).

I did get some days off entirely, but not necessarily weekends. This was my serious introduction to the unnecessarily dangerous, sleep-deprived training for doctors, which is traditional. Internship was just as grueling, as are most residency programs.

We treated people for everything that we could. I didn't even think about insurance. We treated people with respiratory infections, abdominal pain, diarrhea, wounds for suturing, and babies to be delivered. Some patients needed to be transferred elsewhere. We would triage people with fractures and surgical conditions, and then send them on ahead by ambulance to another hospital.

It was cold when I was there, often below freezing. There would be ice on the bare tree branches in the mornings, and spectacular orange sunsets. The landscape was all new to me. There was a lot of red rock, with deep canyons like the Canyon de Chelly and tall formations such as the *Three Sisters*. I went to visit these, as well as caves with pictographs, on my days off. The Navajo reservation is the largest of all of the American *Indian* reservations in the US. The Navajo people call themselves the Dineh (*the people*). They have been there for at least six hundred years.

Those two winter months were difficult in some ways. I felt lonely and isolated. I missed my friends, and I was recently married and missed my wife. I didn't really develop friendships in Ganado. I threw myself into my work, which is what was expected of me. I was a very serious student.

It was also a time of learning so much, which was inherently enjoyable, and not just about medicine. Navajo and Hopi history, the Shalako celebration, other customs, a little bit of language. The smell of sagebrush, and of cedar, which was used as fuel for heating and cooking. The taste of Navajo fry bread.

A lot of what I saw made me angry and sad. There was a constant steady erosion of Navajo culture and language. Poverty was rampant. Traditional housing were hogans, which were large round huts made of the ubiquitous red clay, often home to large extended families. They used wood for fuel, and they had a central smoke hole instead of a chimney. There was no running water in a hogan. The economy was based on grazing sheep and growing crops on parched land. There was also beautiful jewelry of silver and turquoise, woven wool blankets, and pottery. What they didn't use for their household, they sold to tourists, which provided a better income than agriculture.

Alcohol, introduced by the colonizers, led to alcoholism. A westernized diet led to obesity and diabetes. Domestic violence and horrible auto accidents were commonplace.

The non-medical staff were largely Navajo. The experienced nurses in New York understood that nurses often had more knowledge of many things medical than doctors-in-training did, so they would sometimes help out by asking questions discreetly, or even by making direct suggestions. In that charade, the decision was still left to the doctors' discretion.

The nurses in Ganado, who were mostly Navajo or Hopi, were less bold. They were unlikely to question the decisions of medical staff. So, following the medical tradition which I had been taught, I was reluctant to admit that I didn't know what to do and reluctant to ask for help.

This led, understandably, to one memorable incident which bordered on medical malpractice on my part, and I'm not proud of it.

Navajo women often delivered their babies at home, with the assistance of lay midwives. But there was also a trend toward going to the hospital for birthing because that was where doctors were thought to practice superior *scientific* medicine, as opposed to inferior *traditional* medicine.

I had observed a number of births up to that point in New York, but I had little hands-on experience. One night, a woman came into Sage Hospital in labor, in the middle of the night. I was there in the delivery room with one nurse. This mother's medical history indicated several successful vaginal births without the need for any intervention. Perhaps it was the noise of her screaming and groaning. Or perhaps it was the appearance of the baby's head stretched tightly against the vaginal lips that led me to feel scared. I was reluctant to call my mentor and wake him up. I decided I could handle the situation. I went ahead and performed an episiotomy, which was a diagonal cut across one side of the vaginal lips to make room for the baby's head. Both the mother and baby turned out fine. The mother was happy with the outcome.

There was still a large wound which I had made. Its edges needed to be sutured securely shut. I was unable to pull the wound edges together effectively. Since the day was dawning by then, I finally called my mentor in for help. He sutured the wound closed, and no one mentioned the incident afterward. I don't remember seeing the mom for follow-up care—I don't know whether she had any follow-up care. I don't blame myself for my actions at that time because the culture of the medical system had set me up for this problem, but I wish that I had allowed myself to admit that I was scared and that I could have used some help and needed some guidance right at that time.

A few months later, I graduated from medical school. The formal ceremony had a medieval feel to it, with red and black robes draped loosely over our shoulders, and soft square velvet caps on our heads. We tossed the hats awkwardly into the air, finally releasing the pressure of the past four years. And I received a diploma.

I was Eric Lessinger, MD!

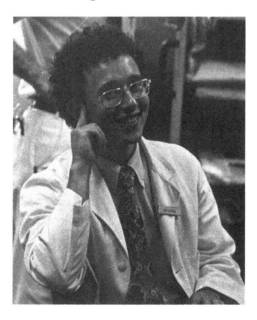

My NYU Med School '72 yearbook photo

Internship year — Lincoln Hospital

Shortly before graduation, most students go through an anxiety-filled process which culminates in *match day*. They apply to a number of hospitals for an internship position. There they would get to be hired as MDs, getting paid for their work for the first time. After successfully completing the internship year, they could begin to practice medicine, after passing another national licensing exam.

I skipped *match day* by applying to one hospital only, where I knew ahead of time that a position would be waiting for me. That was Lincoln Hospital, a municipal hospital in the South Bronx. I arrived there in July 1972. I still felt that time was on our side, that large-scale progressive social change was possible, if not imminent.

When I arrived, there was already a large group of doctors as well as allied health personnel who had formed the *Lincoln Collective*. Calling it a *collective* seemed like the revolutionary thing to do, even though there was nothing particularly collective about it. There was also a revolutionary Puerto Rican party called the Young Lords, who were active in the South Bronx. They were affiliated with the Black Panther Party, and they followed the fashion of the Panthers. They wore purple berets, and they marched in military formation. One thing that they did not do was to carry shotguns in public. Many of the Black Panthers were assassinated by police, but as far as I can recall, no young lords met that fate.

The one year I spent at Lincoln was hugely significant to my personal and medical development. The head of the Department of Pediatrics, Dr. Helen Rodriguez-Trias, was at least loosely affiliated with the Lincoln Collective. And the head of the Department of Medicine was also sympathetic. The collective doctors were leaders with a progressive agenda, and many still are leaders, in Physicians for a National Health Program (PNHP), or in the Medical Committee for Human Rights (MCHR). We're still advocating for single-payer, universal health care, fifty years later. (Essentially what is now called Medicare for All.)

I didn't want to become a specialist, even in the broad field of adult medicine (internal medicine). I didn't want to give up caring for children as well. At Lincoln, I was able to craft my own internship program: nine months of internal medicine and three months of pediatrics.

Section 4: MEDICAL PRACTICE

Rochester, New York
Highland Hospital
Westside Family Health Services

By the end of my internship year, my marriage to Ellen was over. We knew that we would not be making our next move together. After my internship, I was eager to get my license and begin medical practice. I made inquiries and searched in the back of medical journals, looking for a place to begin practice, and I found a job listing in Rochester, New York. Rochester was a city of fewer than one million people. I had a lot of green space in it. There was an annual lilac festival in the spring. And it was surrounded by suburban towns. It appeared quite lovely.

The job offer was at a group of three health centers called Westside. Community health centers seemed like a good fit for me, to *serve the people*, and, as my father had counseled me, to do something useful that needed doing. One site there was in a largely Puerto Rican neighborhood. As I had done in the South Bronx, I could use my rudimentary medical Spanish.

Dr. Michael Klein was the medical director of Westside Health Services, and furthermore, he expressed a distinctly progressive medical agenda for a doctor in a responsible position. I was pleased that he offered me my first job, which I accepted. I moved from Manhattan to Rochester, to rent an apartment and to live alone for the first time in my life. At Westside, there were teams who worked closely and consulted together. We also socialized some. There were six or eight MDs there working at the three centers. Two were women. One was Linda Farley, the wife of Gene Farley, Chairman of the Department of Family Medicine. The other was Susan Soboroff, from Chicago, Radcliffe 1967, who was single. We gradually grew closer, developed a romantic relationship, and with a little encouragement from the rest of the staff, we got married in 1977.

Although I had started working directly after my internship year, I knew that it would make sense for me to get further training, as a resident. At about that time, family practice, as distinct from general practice, was just becoming accepted as a medical specialty in its own right. Dr. Eugene Farley was a pioneer in helping to establish family practice. Dr. Farley was the chairman of the Department of Family Medicine at Highland Hospital, affiliated with the University of Rochester. Once again, I had the good fortune and good timing to be allowed to pursue residency training while continuing to work part-time at Westside.

Trumansburg, New York

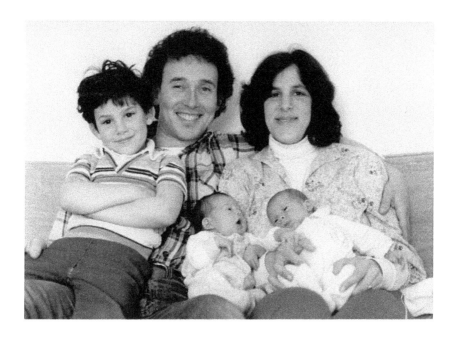

When Susan and I were ready to move on, we searched the medical journals, looking for a practice where we could work as partners. We found it in Trumansburg, New York, a village of about 1700 people 10 miles north of Ithaca, where a GP, Dr. Stanley Gutelius, was planning to retire.

Dr. Gutelius was happy just to have some continuity for his patients. As I recall, he *sold the practice* for little more than the price of the office furniture. He and his wife, who was also his nurse, had a house next to his office, which they rented to us.

The access to our new office was far from compliant with the Americans With Disabilities Act (ADA). There was a full flight of stairs up to the office!

We decided to stay in this little, mostly rural village, and started looking for a house which we could buy. We purchased a large four-bedroom house on the edge of the village, with seven acres of land, and we had a pond dug there. Life at home and at the office was good. We had three children. David was born in 1977 and our twins, Eva and Jesse, were born in 1983.

I added to my FP qualifications, first as a geriatrician and later adding hospice and palliative care. I worked part-time in hospice starting in 1986 and exclusively in hospice as the medical director of Hospicare in Ithaca from 2002 until my retirement in 2014. Our life in the office and at home had been good. Our practice grew and thrived.

We had moved to a larger office with six exam rooms. We hired an RN as well as a secretary. Soon we were joined by medical partners, one at a time—Drs. Joyce Leslie, Suzanne Anderson, John Cooke, Maura McCauley, and Michelle Blegen. Two of the partners found themselves very soon in the middle of nasty, prolonged divorces. Although I didn't realize it at the time, we had many stressors of our own which would lead to the end of our marriage. I got certified as a

family practitioner after two years of residency training following one year of internship. Susan did just
one year of internship, never taking a residency position. She was a good doctor, and her patients didn't
know about her shorter training. Many of her female
patients preferred seeing a female physician. However,
I couldn't help but speculate that she felt overshadowed by me. When I got certified in hospice and palliative care, I would fly to hotels in New Orleans or
Kansas City where the AAHPM would host weeklong
conventions for us to participate in, and network and
dine at the hotels. A hospice NP and I would usually
attend, but Susan wouldn't come along for the ride.

After Susan had finished nursing our children
and returned to work each time, we shared the child
care and cooking as equitably as we could. Neither
of us could provide day care until our three children
were able to come and go on a school bus by themselves. They had a loving day care provider, but I
can't help wondering whether the decision that each
of our children made to work in a field other than
medicine had something to do with the lives which
we modeled for them. Susan and I drifted apart.
When the kids were grown, we went through a difficult divorce. The medical practice which we built,
however, the Trumansburg Family Health Center,
continues to this day, in 2021.

Finding Re-evaluation Counseling (RC)

In this memoir, I have written of two major influences which shaped me from early on in my life, which helped me to become the doctor and the man who I am. Firstly, to heal and repair the world. Secondly, that no one should be able to acquire a fortune by profiting from the work of others, and that everyone who was capable of working should do productive work.

As a young adult, early in my career as a doctor, I came to some important realizations, which built upon the earlier values. All of us are a part of the world which needs healing. Doctors are workers who are highly trained, generally well-respected, and generally do useful work, but we can also use some help, if we are willing to accept it.

At the end of my internship year in mid-1973, Ellen and I had a relatively amicable divorce (no assets, no fault, no lawyer). I found a job in Rochester and went to work, and I enjoyed that. However, I had never lived alone before, and that felt difficult. I started to see the psychologist at the health center where I worked. He was only slightly older than I, and very open about his feelings. Our relationship felt collegial. He too had recently divorced. He and I decided to end the formal counseling relationship, and to join a men's group instead. Once there, we felt safe to talk about anything we wanted to, and it is fair to say that since we were all heterosexual men, a lot of the talk was about women.

In 1973, I was about twenty-five years old, and my psychologist friend told me about a public talk being given in Rochester by a man named Harvey Jackins. His talk was called an "Introduction to Re-Evaluation Counseling." Harvey was about the same age as my father. He and my father had a lot in common, as I saw it. They both rejected the cap-italist system. They thought that, at this stage of human development, we could do a lot better. My father was an openly communist Jew in New York; Harvey sounded like a communist. He had been a member of the International Workers of the World (IWW) in the Northwestern US.

But Harvey was also very animated. He seemed both relaxed and intense and at the same time self-confident. He made eye contact with many people, including me, and he seemed pleased with me as well as with himself.

Most striking of all, he talked about this theory of behavior that he had stumbled upon, and how he had developed and tested it. He had a logical mind. He noticed that after a person had a chance to vent, say, like having a good cry, that person seemed to

ERIC LESSINGER, MD

be able to think more clearly. From there, with many more steps in between, he went on to believe that people get hurt in many ways, and that when they don't get a chance to vent enough (by crying, shaking, laughing, shouting, etc.), they are left with some part of the hurt, which leaves them unable to think rationally.

This theory seemed plausible, although maybe a little too oversimplified to explain the mysteries of human brains, with all our feelings and thoughts.

I was excited by what I had heard and seen and felt that evening. I wrote a letter to my father about it, and I included a short pamphlet which explained the basics of the theory. After a few days, my father wrote out a reply, with a fountain pen, in his fine, elegant script. He explained in very deliberate and analytic prose, including some references to Freud and Adler, which he used for comparison, to explain why this *Jackins fellow* was wrong. Well, that took the wind out of my sails. My father, who had been my mentor and my hero, didn't see the possibility that this theory might be accurate.

I persisted in trying to make sense of all this. My father and Harvey seemed to agree about so much which was important—the potential for human-ity to create a better world, the need for collective action by the working class, the need to end racism in the US, etc. And then, I had a new thought—Harvey had been able to find the piece that seemed to be missing from my father's worldview, about both feeling and thinking. Harvey made a sharp distinction between thinking and feeling, but he also saw a key connection between them.

I wasn't ready to jump in with both feet. Re-evaluation Counseling, or simply RC, was what Harvey named the process and organization he had created. I was skeptical; it just seemed overly simplistic, overly optimistic, and unrealistic. For example, Harvey believed that all people were good. Thinking about monsters like Adolf Hitler, I found the notion of Hitler's goodness hard to swallow. I thought that RC was not likely to be able to really deliver on its promises.

This began a period of serious reflection for me. I felt torn between Harvey and my father. At age twenty-five, I was an independent adult. I didn't need a father figure. What I was seeking was a belief system, or at least a theory, which would make sense to me.

I had known my father for twenty-five years; I had just met Harvey Jackins. I loved my father, and several times he had said, "No matter what you do, and no matter how badly you think you have behaved, your mother and I will always love you." He was a hero to me.

Harvey Jackins was an enigma to me, very different from my father. As I had noticed when I met him, he appeared to be relaxed but animated, and very self-confident. I wasn't sure that I knew anyone who had all of those qualities. He seemed incautious, and he could appear almost fierce at times. In retrospect, I also realized that I knew very few Jews who had all those qualities.

RC actually helped me to reclaim my somewhat atrophied Judaism. Harvey was not a Jew, but he had a great deal of respect for Jewish tradition. Most importantly, he recognized a pattern of hurt among Jews which caused us to feel that we had no allies and could count only on ourselves. He asked us Jews to treat *everyone* as a potential ally, despite our fears. Conversely, non-Jews often felt that they couldn't really get close to Jews and that our ritual practices were a mystery. So RC instituted a plan to demystify that, by celebrating Shabbat for everyone on Friday night, at the beginning of a weekend workshop.

I went through a very deliberate and conscious process, to decide whether I was going to follow Harvey's thinking or my father's.

I tested Re-Evaluation Counseling, talking with people who had joined the group. More importantly, I tried out the process of exchanging time, or co-counseling. It did seem to *work*. That is, I felt better after I had a session, and more importantly, I was able to think more clearly afterward.

I thought Harvey probably did have the piece that was missing from my father's understanding of people. With some trepidation and some sadness, I made the conscious choice to follow Harvey Jackins instead of continuing to rely upon my father. Within a month or two, I signed up to take a class in the Fundamentals of Co-Counseling.

There are many key points to make about the theory and practice of RC. (However, the only way to get a full understanding of it is to be a part of it.)

We take turns, working in pairs, on an equal footing. There is no therapist/client relationship. First, both people focus solely on only one of us; thinking, feeling, crying, and laughing; trying to unravel our hurts; then we switch roles.

RC has a *one-point program*, which is to use this process to recover our best thinking and to assist others to do the same. We encourage people to think broadly, without limits. We are constantly testing our theory, by holding it up to the light of *discharge*, which is what we call those various processes of crying, laughing, yawning, trembling, raging, etc.

Over the course of years, we have amassed a large volume of literature: books by Harvey Jackins, periodicals for many constituency groups, and pamphlets.

Sometimes we develop policies which we have agreed upon. Every policy is labeled a *draft policy*, subject to change, based upon re-evaluated clearer thinking. Many examples of policies regard liberation issues, such as for women, blacks, and Jews. There are also guidelines, which have been adopted over the years, by a meeting once every four years of the entire worldwide leadership.

There are only a few actual rules or requirements. The rule that many people seem to have the most trouble with is the *no-socializing* rule. This means that outside of RC, we do not establish romantic, business, or other relationships with other co-counselors.

Another rule is to maintain confidentiality, especially about the identity of a *client*, and about what he/she might have said in a co-counseling session. Even referring to the *material* of the agreed-upon client can be hurtful, or *restimulating* to them.

RC is a hierarchical organization, but it is not autocratic. Each level of leadership is carefully vetted by the level above it. There are certified teachers of RC, *reference* people for geographical areas, then for whole geographic regions, etc.

What may be the most impressive to me about RC are the ways in which the organization has grown and developed since I joined it many years ago. At first, it attracted mostly college students, mostly white and middle class, who often attended colleges known to be liberal. There were more women than men (this hasn't changed). Jews were over-represented compared to our population. It started in the US, and the only language written or spoken was English.

Most of us were attracted to Harvey's left-leaning ideas but were largely focused on using the process to improve our own lives. And from the very beginning, it also became clear that every one of us is oppressed in some way. Women are oppressed; males dominate. Men are oppressed as well, but not by women. Rather it is the structure of the expectations in our societies themselves that are oppressive. Typically, men have done heavier and more dangerous work and are expected to be tough. Everyone also internalizes their oppression to some extent. And we all seek liberation from oppression.

People from all social classes, races, and religions can become attracted to RC. People who come from loving families or from abusive families can become attracted to RC. And there are several key issues that must be dealt with expeditiously. Racism is often deadly, especially against people of African Heritage in the US due to the legacy of four hundred years of slavery. The climate emergency, which is a ticking time bomb. And the oppressive system of capitalism which is careening out of control.

The RC organization has gradually been implementing changes. These reflect a movement away from the US as the dominant voice and English as the dominant language. Non-white people are taking more leadership at all levels. There is RC activity in dozens of countries, including Africa, Asia, and the global south. and literature in dozens of languages. *Re-evaluation* is really happening in RC.

I will admit that there have been times when I felt upset by something in RC. It seemed too good to be true, or I was naïve. Or that someone in a position of leadership was not treating me well. (That can happen—people sometimes make mistakes). I never completely broke with the organization, however. I still think that RC provides an excellent framework for understanding what is happening in our world, and for our liberation.

My breakdown

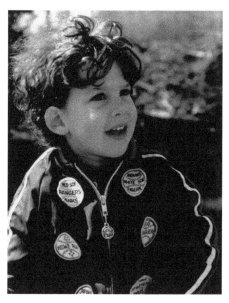

"What's wrong, Papa?"

In my own life and in my medical practice, I have experienced some physical injuries (which have usually resolved quickly) and some emotional hurts, some of which have had lingering effects. I came to realize that everyone in our society gets hurt often severely and that sometimes they suffer lingering effects. The contents of those hurts, however, are unique to each individual.

From early on in medical practice, I was able to listen well to patients most of the time. As time went on, I got more comfortable with people of all sorts.

When someone's voice started to crack, I would try to relax within myself. If they started to cry, I would not try to distract them—just the opposite. I discovered that "a good cry" can be helpful to me and to others. Other people thought that I "had it together." I must admit that I thought so too. I was a successful family doctor at the height of my career. But I thought I was learning that even those people who didn't appear to "have it together" might not be as "crazy" as they appeared to be. If I could listen closely to what they were saying, sometimes I could help them sort out their thoughts, and then they often made sense.

So my family and friends were surprised and shocked when seemingly out of the blue, I no longer seemed to "have it together" but rather seemed to be acting "crazy"!

It was 1981. I was thirty-one years old, active, and full of energy. In addition to having an active and growing medical practice, I went mountain biking with a group of friends. Susan and I had a three-year-old son at home.

The village of Trumansburg was almost entirely Christian. The only other doctor in town was Christian. Susan and I were both Jews, but her family was more observant. I had been raised in an entirely secular environment. But now, in this overwhelmingly Christian environment, I started to learn more about Judaism, explore Jewish history, and acknowledge more fully my undeniable connection to my people.

When I was born, the world had only recently learned about the horrors of the Nazi holocaust. After surviving centuries of intermittent anti-Semitism, we were faced with a monstrous leader who offered his people a "final solution" to the "Jewish problem." Until then, I was able to keep the terror of the Holocaust at bay. I had been insulated and "protected" from this knowledge. My family had told me that we didn't know of anybody in our family who had been lost in the Holocaust. (Many had come here to the US, and some had gone to the USSR, but my family had lost touch with whomever else might be left in the rest of Europe.)

I allowed myself for the first time to acknowledge and feel the horror. In retrospect, I see this as unfortunate, for two reasons.

Firstly, it led to my own "breakdown," which I will describe. Secondly, it led to what I consider to be an unhealthy preoccupation with what happened in the Holocaust not because it didn't happen but because it left so many Jews able to see themselves only as victims. They invoke the defensive slogan "Never Again," which I think has made it difficult for some Jews to acknowledge that we also act oppressively sometimes.

I thought about the Holocaust, and I started to take it seriously. The more I thought about it, the more terrified I felt. I became preoccupied. I felt like I was living in it. And then it was as if I flipped a switch, and I realized that the Nazi Holocaust was actually over. At the same time, I was still terrified, but I denied it. This was not particularly rational, but I could not recognize the contradiction there. My terror felt like it had turned into joy overnight, and I wanted to tell everybody the good news. This puzzled the people who knew me. I was in an excited state, and nothing they could do seemed to slow me down. I hardly slept. I ate very little. I couldn't go back to work. People became frightened. I became increasingly incoherent and paranoid from lack of sleep. My wife was scared. She had never seen me this way before. On the other hand, our three-year-old son was not scared. He just asked, "What's wrong, Papa?"

Finally, my wife called an ambulance, and I was transported thirty miles or more to the nearest inpatient psychiatric unit, which was in Syracuse. By that time, my relationship with present-time reality had become very tenuous. (I was "psychotic.") I felt terrified and paranoid, and I remember that I

actually tried to punch one of the ambulance atten-
dants, so they made sure that I was kept in restraints
for the rest of the trip.

When I arrived at the unit, my wife debriefed
the staff, while I was quickly injected with a strong
sedative, a "first generation" antipsychotic drug,
Haldol. But according to my discharge summary, I
was still "quite agitated and non-responsive to ver-
bal suggestion," so I was put in seclusion to decrease
my overloaded stimulation and sensory input. I
slept for the first time in days. I may have slept for
twenty-four hours straight. I probably missed two
or three days of my life, in a haze, in and out of
awareness. I was initially unable to communicate
effectively. The psychiatrist supervising my case saw
me daily, but I'm not sure how long our visits were.
He also wrote in my discharge summary that I didn't
recognize him on our first few visits. Still, he kept
me sedated. I continued to have an inflated sense of
my own power. I was also very scared, and I felt like
I was fighting for my life. I was anything but pow-
erful in relation to the psychiatrist, who decided
everything for me, including when he thought that
I was sufficiently in control of myself again to be
freed. All the rest of that brief week was fuzzy. He
switched me to oral tablets of Haldol to take four
times a day, and I was still sedated. However, there

was one bright spot. A hospital aide, an older Black man named Robert, said two things that struck me as helpful and wise: "We're all on the right string. It's just that we yo-yo different." "That's what life is about. There's no book on *you*." At that point, I was allowed a pencil and paper, so I wrote down those quotes.

My wife drove up to visit. I was eager to leave the hospital. When she saw me, I was far from rational. But she was no longer scared of me or of my physical state, which was not yet healthy. However, I seemed sufficiently recognizable as the person she knew that she was willing to sign me out "against advice" after just five days of being locked up. The psychiatrist warned us that there was a risk of "loss of control." She brought me home, and "loss of control" did not happen. I agreed to keep taking some sedative drugs, and I slept better at home. What also happened was that I felt very ashamed of what I had done—a respected young physician (who seemed to "have it together") became very out of touch with reality. I came crashing down from my high. I went to see an outpatient psychiatrist in Ithaca for six weeks. He had me take an antidepressant drug. This also blunted my feelings, but it allowed me to find my way back to my previous good health. I felt better after six weeks. I've never looked back with regret. I've never been depressed again.

A lot of what I couldn't remember came from the discharge summary written by my inpatient psychiatrist. He had a fairly accurate description of my past and recent history. His description of my time in the hospital seemed to reflect his perceptions honestly. Most importantly, and to his credit, he did not assume that he could label me with a psychiatric diagnosis. Instead, he wrote:

> Final diagnosis: "Delirium of unknown etiology."
> Condition on discharge: "Good."
> Prognosis: "Good."

Hospice and palliative care

As I progressed in my own learning, I found that I enjoyed teaching and that I was good at it. Whenever I reached the point at which I thought that I had something to offer, I did. I worked closely with nurse practitioners in various capacities, and in those situations, I usually had something to share, but also sometimes something to learn as well, often because the nurses were mostly female. While I was in my residency at Highland Hospital in Rochester, I was able to teach interns, and to share information with my fellow residents. In my medical practice, I exchanged information with my partners and colleagues. And although Cayuga Medical Center was not a teaching hospital, I did take the opportunity, as the only hospice physician in the area, to give a PowerPoint presentation to the medical staff. And just as I had done by taking a six-week elective on the Navajo reservation, so there was a fourth-year medical student who shadowed me for five weeks, as I did my job as a hospice doctor, in the Cayuga Medical Center ICU and at the Hospicare residence. I saved a personal note from her.

It read:

Dear Dr. Lessinger (October 31, 2013)

It was a real pleasure being your student these past five weeks. Even though it was a short time, it gave me a better sense of what comfort care is all about, and how to communicate with the patients and family on such a difficult topic. From watching your interactions and discussing assessments, it was very clear to me how much patients appreciate and need your service and insight. Also, I really appreciate the small gestures of giving me articles to read, showing that you care. Best wishes on your upcoming retirement—Hospicare has some big shoes to fill—thanks again for your time and caring.

Warmest, E___

I became a geriatrician as a natural progression from my family practice, with a panel of largely older patients. It was then also a natural progression to hospice and palliative care, after presiding over many deaths which were foreseeable but not preventable.

Dame Cecily Saunders had brought the modern hospice movement from England to the US in the mid-1970s. Elisabeth Kübler-Ross' work *On Death and Dying*, which elucidates five stages of grief, became a best-seller, at least among my cohort. The AFP had developed a curriculum which led to a Certificate of Additional Qualifications in Hospice and Palliative Care. A hospice program had just started up in Ithaca, with one multidisciplinary team. They needed to expand, so I became the head of a second multidisciplinary team there.

Up until that time, care for dying patients had been provided in the home, which was clearly the best choice when feasible, or in facilities such as nursing homes when necessary. Then a group of people in Ithaca developed the idea of building a dedicated residential facility, which could provide hospice care when, for whatever reason, care could no longer be provided at home. The idea was to provide a very professional and welcoming, but also homelike situation. Funds were easily raised for the construction of a six-bed unit, which opened in 1995, and which later grew to twelve beds as the need increased. I became medical director of the newly named "Hospicare" in 2002, and I worked there until my retirement in 2014. During that time, I was employed by Hospicare, and my only job at the Trumansburg office was as an informal teacher/consultant.

Palliation refers to reducing symptoms without curing the underlying disease. Think about that. It is not usually a simple decision for a patient or a medical provider. It may mean that there is currently no known cure (although there may be a cure on the horizon). It probably means that both the patient and the doctor agree that no matter what the cause of the disease is, the pain or other symptoms themselves are severe enough to demand treatment. Such treatment can usually be effective, but there may be times when the side effects give you pause ("the treatment is worse than the disease"). These decisions cannot be made without clarifying one's beliefs, goals, priorities, pain tolerance, family relationships, etc. One of the most important functions of the doctor or nurse practitioner (as well as of the entire palliative care team) is to help with this clarifying process, without imposing the team's beliefs upon the patient.

Most often, a patient opting for palliative care is a cognitively aware, mentally competent, and autonomously functioning adult. Hopefully all adults, but especially older adults, will have the foresight to fill out a will, a living will, a medical power of attorney, and instructions to their family and their physicians expressing their wishes regarding resuscitation. A "Do-Not-Resuscitate" (DNR) order written by the patient, describing the circumstances in which they would choose not to be resuscitated, can be very helpful to the doctor and the family (e.g., "If I am declared *brain dead*, with no hope of recovery, do not attempt resuscitation"). Even so, there may be conflict, when different family members hold different beliefs, or when they have different interpretations of the patient's expressed wishes. When a patient enrolls in hospice, a DNR order should be routine.

When a patient enrolls in hospice, the hospice doctor certifies that the patient is not expected to live more than six months, and the patient and family agree that all treatment should be directed toward comfort; that treatment directed toward a cure is not appropriate. But even in palliative care, these issues and these decisions can be difficult.

There are times when a parent or guardian must make decisions for someone else. When one or more family members become involved, the issues often multiply. It is generally a good idea to keep the doctor's beliefs out of the equation, but it may be important to provide information and to help the patient and/or family with decision-making. Fear, depression, or ignorance (or any distortion of the ability to be rational) has sometimes required me to provide more direct information and guidance. That feels like an awesome responsibility, more or less substituting my judgment for that of the person whose moral and legally specified responsibility it is to make the decision. Still, I found that it was more often rewarded with gratitude from patients and families rather than with unhappiness or resentment.

The line between hospice and palliative care can become blurred at times. In hospice, the disease is believed to be terminal, and death is predicted to occur within six months or less (if the disease follows its usual course). Without a crystal ball, such predictions cannot be correct 100 percent of the time. The current federal regulations in this country require that the physician, who is the head of the team, certifies by a signature that the patient has a life expectancy of six months or less. If another six months pass and the patient is still alive, the certification can be renewed for one more six-month period. Occasionally, a patient can be discharged from hospice services, although they are likely to remain on palliative care, given their diagnosis.

One of the challenges which I faced many times was when a patient himself was severely ill and unable to speak, and the family member who was assigned the role of speaking as the proxy for the patient would tell me, "Do everything you can, Doc!" The implication was that they wanted the patient to stay alive as long as possible. Then in some way or another, I had to ask, "Just what does that mean?" If unconscious, can we gauge the amount of suffering or pain they are experiencing? Should I be instructed to give only as much pain relief as will allow them to moan but not speak? These are real questions, which have to be asked compassionately. Asking such questions got easier over time, but they still made me uneasy, and glad that I'm clear about what I want when I die. My family should have minimal angst about what they decide.

The ultimate difficulty comes when the proxy just can't let go, and he or she wants me to attempt resuscitation if and when the heart stops. I would not do this to a terminal patient. I may have once or twice gone through the motions of a *code*, when I thought that there was still enough time for the proxy to be present at that mysterious moment when the patient slips from being alive to being dead, or as some would say, moves from this world to the next.

A vignette has stayed with me from my work as a hospice physician, while in the ICU of the Ithaca hospital. It is a fond memory (and it is easier to remember in detail because I preserved a thank you card which the family sent to me). I was caring for several generations of an African-American family. I knew the elderly patriarch of this family for only a few days before he died, in a coma. The family had some difficulty letting him go. (And I must admit that some black families have some mistrust of white doctors, who, they feel, don't care as much, or work as hard as they could, to treat their families.) That was not the case with this family.

It turned out that a daughter of the patriarch fell ill, and also was cared for in the ICU. She had many children, and I had multiple family meetings with them in a conference room adjacent to the ICU. They were devout Christians, and they knew that I was a Jew. They may also have been aware, as was I, that there is a solid Old Testament connection between Jews and Black Christians in this country (e.g., through spirituals and slave songs, and in the fight for social justice).

Because there were so many people in that third generation of the family, they appointed one of the sisters as the spokesperson. They would confer with each other about how to proceed, and then several of them would meet with me. We related to each other in very human ways—I was respectful of them, and they were not over-awed by me. And somewhere along the line, they started calling me "Smokey." I was amused and pleased, and in a way, honored, that they noticed that I actually had kinky hair, a kindly face, and hazel-colored eyes; I looked a lot like Smokey Robinson, a very popular Motown singer of those times, who was also my contemporary. Their mother ultimately had a peaceful death.

On the card which I received from them, there was a short poem printed on the front entitled "Your Thoughtfulness Is a Reflection of God's Love." Printed on the inside, "Your thoughtfulness meant much more than any words can say. Thank you very much." The hand-written note which was enclosed read:

"Dear Smokey,

We appreciate all you have done and been to our family and our mother through her last weeks. You are a great man, and the P___ family loves you and wants to thank you for taking such great care of our loved one in her last stages. Sorry, this is so late, but we couldn't go on without letting you know how much we appreciate you!

With lots of love,

J_____ and the P____ family

P.S. We love you Smokey, and thank you from the bottom of our hearts."

Conclusion

In this memoir, I have tried to be unflinchingly honest and fair, neither minimizing nor romanticizing its significance. I think I have reason to be pleased with myself. I also know that I am not able to think or act as rationally as I would like, and I believe that I will always want to continue the pursuit of my personal healing.

It is becoming increasingly obvious that our planet too needs healing. All humans on this planet are now living in societies in need of healing. And without becoming alarmist or panicked or paralyzed, we can notice that there is some urgency to bring about change.

The COVID-19 pandemic has been devastating to life recently, leading to more than five million deaths worldwide as of 2022, and causing the fraying of our social fabric, but this pandemic will probably not become permanent. On the other hand, the global climate emergency needs coordinated effective action before it is too late, if humans are to survive.

And it seems that with every crisis, the gaps widen between the rich and poor, between the white people and the people of the global majority, and between the so-called developed nations (advanced capitalist countries) and the so-called third world, who are poor or colonized or both. This situation is oppressive and deadly.

I have never stopped wanting things to be right. I will continue to work with other "white" people to end racism. (Actually, most of us are some shade of *pink* rather than *white*. Notice that in common parlance, white is associated with good and black with evil). I will continue to work with people of all social classes to end the gulf which separates the people who produce the goods and services from the people who *own* them.

I remain optimistic. Helping people is what I do. However, I'm not going to sacrifice myself in the process. One important thing that I am learning is that when I am with other people who love me and who can think well about me, it serves me well to relax and be vulnerable. Then I can laugh, cry, and heal.

I want to share widely what I have learned with as many people as possible. I'm still alive. And I'm looking forward to the next chapter!

The End

ABOUT THE AUTHOR

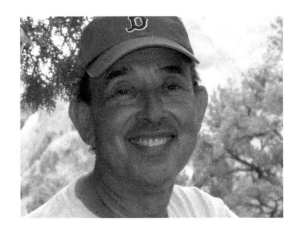

Eric Lessinger, MD, grew up in Brooklyn, New York. He is a family doctor who graduated from NYU Medical School in 1972 and did his internship at Lincoln Hospital in the South Bronx, New York, and his residency training in Rochester, New York. He practiced family medicine and hospice care in Trumansburg, New York, near Ithaca, for many years. He is now happily retired and lives in Gloucester, Massachusetts, with his wife Meredith and their two cats.

Printed in the USA
CPSIA information can be obtained
at www.ICGtesting.com
LVHW061053200624
783566LV00017B/468